WE'RE PREGNANT!

D0012787

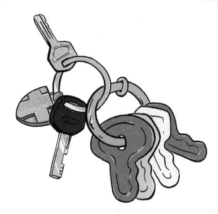

WE'RE PREGNANT!

The First-Time Dad's Pregnancy Handbook

Everything You Need to Know for Your Partner & Baby

ADRIAN KULP

Foreword by Heather B. Armstrong,
creator of *dooce*®

Illustrations by Jeremy Nguyen

**ROCKRIDGE
PRESS**

For general information on our other products and services or to obtain technical support,
please contact our Customer Care Department within the United States at (866) 744-2665,
or outside the United States at (510) 253-0500.

Rockridge Press publishes its books in a variety of electronic and print formats. Some
content that appears in print may not be available in electronic books, and vice versa.

TRADEMARKS: Rockridge Press and the Rockridge Press logo are trademarks or registered
trademarks of Callisto Media Inc. and/or its affiliates, in the United States and other
countries, and may not be used without written permission. All other trademarks are the
property of their respective owners. Rockridge Press is not associated with any product
or vendor mentioned in this book.

Illustrations © Jeremy Nguyen, 2018
Icons © Megan Dailey, 2018

ISBN: Print 978-1-93975-468-4 | eBook 978-1-93975-469-1

*For Ava, Charlie, Mason, and the
next little one for whom we wait with
open arms—you are my life, my love,
and my reason for being.*

I hope I make you proud.

Contents

Foreword

Finding out that you're going to be a first-time parent is simultaneously a terrifying experience and the most profound opportunity to evolve as a human. I have two children, both daughters. My then husband and I planned each pregnancy, but our approach toward the nine-month process was somewhat different. While I devoured every book about pregnancy and the first year of parenthood, he was less enthralled with the logistics and trusted that he would fulfill his role more organically. Men who are truly interested in becoming reliable partners and fathers should be committed to the well-being of their family from the very beginning. When you see those double lines on that pregnancy test, what's important to your partner should be just as important to you.

Even though women continue to break glass ceilings—filling high profile CEO positions and running for president of the free world—the undeniable fact remains that women are still expected to take on the majority of childcare. More often than not, whether they are staying at home or working as the breadwinners, mothers will eventually take on most of the responsibility of their children. For me, this imbalance took a heavy toll, both physically and mentally. It also took a toll on my marriage. Shortly after the birth of my first daughter, I found myself feeling profoundly alone—with the baby, with my thoughts, with the physical task of taking care of her every need—and soon I succumbed to crippling panic attacks.

I frequently called my husband at work and pleaded with him to come home. Sometimes I called him just to hear the voice of another adult. My panic attacks became so severe that when my daughter was six months old, I checked myself into a hospital. I would have given anything to feel less alone.

Women are pressured to balance it all, but if anything, the resounding message from the massive growth of the community around my website dooce® is that moms need support—physical, emotional, and psychological. Even though both parents are figuring it all out as everything unfolds, more often than not that road is lonelier for the mother, even if there is a father in the picture. And, despite strong customs, cultures, or traditions that thrive on this imbalance, mothers shouldn't have to bear the majority of the stress and the grinding minutiae of raising children. Mothers shouldn't have to justify why they need their partners in the trenches alongside them.

Adrian Kulp recognized his responsibility as a father and as a partner early during his wife's first pregnancy. In *We're Pregnant! The First-Time Dad's Pregnancy Handbook*, Adrian shares the life-changing and life-saving lessons that helped him thrive, and he provides guidance tailored specifically for first-time dads. He delivers the right balance of clinical information and ways to support expecting moms, all while speaking to what men need to hear in a way that will make sense to them and their roles as fathers. Writing and coaching as a once clueless and misguided first-time dad, Adrian clearly understands the challenges ahead and makes it his mission to get first-time dads to start maturing, to pay attention, and most importantly to understand what it means to provide support.

As a practical handbook, this book is straightforward and offers small and memorable bites of insight. It focuses on weekly pregnancy milestones so that the father can stay on track with the mother and the baby's developments throughout those nine months and that "fourth trimester." This book also offers weekly to-do lists that address the mother's specific needs. Boyfriends, husbands, partners, and even second-time fathers who may need a refresher will benefit from this book as they learn to communicate better, become more proactive, and increase their level of empathy for the person who statistically is stuck with all the heavy lifting.

Heather B. Armstrong, creator of dooce®

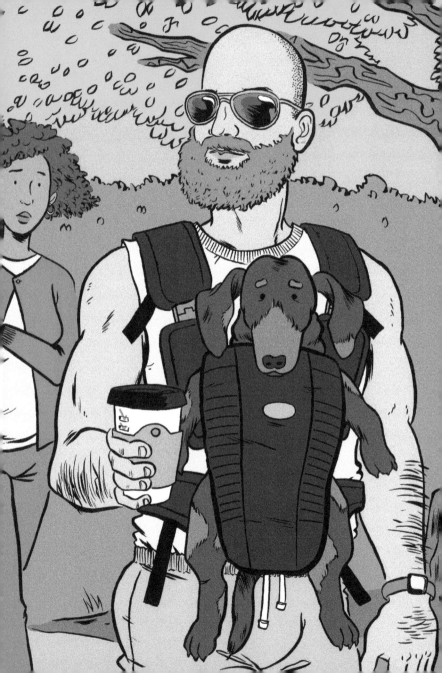

So You're Going to Be a Dad . . .

First off, congratulations, high fives, and down lows for having the insight, inspiration, and love that propelled you to pick up this book. Whether you read this book while commuting to work on the subway, taking a coffee break, or relaxing at home with a frosty beverage after everyone's gone to bed, it will be worth your while. You're about to become a father—and there's no bigger or more exciting thing on this earth. You have the awesome responsibility of shaping a young mind and becoming the role model that your child is going to need well past adolescence and maybe even into their own parenthood. Being a father is life changing on so many levels. Take it from me; I'm a father of three with the fourth on the way. Yes, I'm exhausted, but being 100 percent invested trumps any purported downsides.

Learning that you will be a dad for the first time may be accompanied by overwhelming feelings of anxiety and fear—but that's normal. I went through it, as do most dads. These fears kick *every* new dad right in the gut with a pair of soccer cleats. Will I suck at this? What if I screw up? What if I drop the baby? What if I forget the car seat on top of the car and start driving?

I openly admit that I wasn't quite ready to take on the responsibilities of being a dad, even though my wife and I were actively trying to get pregnant during our first year of marriage. I was still enjoying the freedoms of the life I had created nearly a decade before we met. Even into the first few months of my marriage, I maintained my previously curated schedule, coming and going as I pleased, with little consideration for my wife and her needs. For better or for worse, I was selfish for so many years, truly caring only about myself and my needs.

So it's not an exaggeration to say that fatherhood caught me by surprise, literally. The first time that those double lines on the pregnancy test made an appearance in my life was in 2008 as I was waking up after a night of debauchery while out on the town with friends. As I lay there, reeking of booze, snoring, and trying not to choke on my own saliva, my wife had placed that positive pregnancy stick on my nightstand. She had taken the test—by herself—the night before, after I'd promised to come home early but then didn't. The curiosity had overwhelmed her, and she took the leap without me. And I don't blame her.

To this day, one of my biggest regrets was not being there to support her and share the emotional reaction. The idea of becoming a father for the first time was frightening, and the notion of what it meant to be a dad just did not register because I didn't know where to begin.

It was 16 weeks later at the corresponding prenatal appointment when I learned that, on top of this new *dad* concept, I was having a daughter. I knew nothing about being a father and never had any sisters growing up, so I knew even less about being a father to a little girl and raising her to become a strong, confident person. The weight of those ultrasound results hit me immediately and all at once.

My wife was equally surprised by the results; home pregnancy tests check for the hCG (human chorionic gonadotropin) hormone; it's in her system if she's pregnant and has missed her period. At the time, though, she didn't necessarily comprehend that it's very rare that someone gets a false positive on a pregnancy test. Yes, you can definitely get false negatives, but it was clear we were most likely expecting our first baby.

Once the reality of the situation settled in, my wife (a full-time working mother-to-be) had embraced her new identity. She was already light-years ahead of me—collecting a slew of pregnancy books, pushing away wine at dinner, and instinctively constructing an internal filter that would serve as a sorting mechanism for every piece of advice that came at her (and they came from all directions: from her mom, my mom, sisters, aunts, friends, colleagues, obstetricians, and even random strangers at the airport).

It's no secret that the stressors and responsibilities of pregnancy and babies fall on women, and when you think about it, it's a bad deal and unfair. Yes, women are built with maternal instincts, but there are many things that your partner wouldn't know without a handy book to tell her what she should be expecting. So the reality is that all of us—both men and women—start off clueless when it comes to pregnancy; the difference is that women have no choice but to push through the unknown. They don't try, they just *do*.

When my wife found out that she was pregnant, she picked up several books to help her navigate through what she didn't know, like how in the hell her body was going to stretch out and make room to support a small human the size of a Thanksgiving turkey and then push the kid out through an opening the size of a keyhole. Of course, this is all on top of visualizing the unimaginable pain from contractions that come in waves, sending out slight and sporadic sensations of discomfort at first but then tripling in seismic intensity and occurring closer together. Or considering the not-that-comforting alternative—a giant epidural needle attached to what looks more like a caulking gun than a syringe inserted into her spinal nerve. And let's not forget vaginal tearing, vaginal stitches, hemorrhoids, and the possibility of a C-section. Talk about stepping up. So a man, a dad-to-be, shouldn't use the fear of the unknown and being clueless as excuses to avoid or shirk his duties.

Instead of sitting back, taking the path of least resistance, and allowing our partner to bear the burden of what is coming our way over the next nine months and beyond, we guys need to lose the "dude" act and learn to be the man that our partners see in us so we can be the kind of dad our children will look up to.

I'll be the first to admit: The path of least resistance feels the easiest and most convenient. While it may pass muster when it comes to minutia like doing only your laundry and skipping hers (because you're not sure how to wash her good underwear and can't be bothered to ask her or learn) or washing your ride so it's clean for the week ahead and leaving hers to look like it was pulled from the bottom of a lake, this is a situation in which that just won't cut it. This is one of the biggest experiences you'll ever have in your lifetime, so get involved and take action.

Among my close friends, I was one of the first to take the plunge (getting married and starting a family), and while I may not have expressed it openly, part of my fear stemmed from worrying about losing the bonds that I'd worked so hard to create with "my boys." But it was time. It was time for me to make the leap into manhood. After having this epiphany, I decided to live life on life's terms and let my fears fall to the wayside. True friends will always find their way back around, and the reality was that I was starting my own family. I decided that no matter how many times we are blessed with the ability to get pregnant (four times now), I'd be there for my wife as much as possible. To this day, I've been fortunate enough to have missed only one doctor's appointment.

It's okay to feel uninformed, even clueless, during this time— hell, I most certainly was. I used this challenging opportunity as something to grab on to, an emotional geodetic survey marker where I could meet to connect with my wife, making us stronger partners. As much as we hate admitting our fears and weaknesses, there's no better time than *now*. My weaknesses heavily outweighed my strengths, but I tried to make up for my missteps and potential embarrassments by owning them and making a note to never do that shit again.

It's scary. You're entering the great wide unknown . . . but you're doing it *together*.

Whether you decided long ago that you will have an active role in this pregnancy or you just came to this realization, over the next many pages, I will make sure that you don't waste time wondering what you can do or could've done to help along the journey.

The mother-to-be is already well on her way to educating herself on what she needs to do, and I will give you everything you need to finish this incredibly transformative adventure together. So lay down your fancy gym shorts, take off the Fitbit, and throw on your Wranglers or Dickies, because we're about to get our hands dirty.

The Whys and Hows

When I decided to focus fully on the pregnancy, albeit 16 weeks late, I immediately turned my attention to the books that my wife had already read and memorized and that were now sitting behind the toilet collecting dust. (I assume that she left those there as a hint for me.)

I was motivated to learn what was happening with her on a physical *and* emotional level so that I could absorb this information and do my part. But after reading the first few chapters of a telephone book–size handbook, I felt frustrated. There was so much information. Some of it was relevant to both parents, but the book was mostly written for Mom. There weren't many things I could use as a first-time dad for practical purposes, for the day to day.

In writing this book, my main goal is not only to spell out what dads can expect as their partners' bellies grow but also point out what *you* can actually do to help support her and your growing family. While it took me almost four months to get up to speed, you can start now. This is a pregnancy action plan for the next 12 months—we can't forget about postpartum—so that you can be involved, engaged, and productive.

Over the past eight years, I've written more than 500 articles for my blog, *Dad or Alive: The Confessions of an Unexpected Stay-at-Home Dad,* which also became the basis for my first book, which was a comedic parenting memoir. The book explores my bumpy transition from full-time TV executive to eventual primary caregiver. I've also written several pieces for *HuffPost Parents, The Bump,* and *Parents* magazine. In 2013, I produced *Modern Dads* for A&E, a show that focused on stay-at-home dads in Austin, Texas. And in early 2017, I took a position as head of creative and branded content for a massive online community called *The Life of Dad.* With all that professional "authority" on fatherhood, as well as being a career dad, you'd think that I would have all my shit together. But life doesn't work that way. Even now as my wife and I are preparing for our fourth kid, I still feel clueless, relearning many things that I thought I had mastered.

Nonetheless, some things still prove to be true, and if I had known these things when I became a first-time dad, life would have been a lot less stressful. But in this former dad-to-be's defense, I didn't even know what I didn't know; I had no clue what questions to even ask. It would have been helpful to have some guidance from dads who've been through the tried-and-true test of fatherhood. That's why I decided to write this book. This book exists because of both the mistakes I made and the lessons I know now but wish I knew at the start of this crazy and wonderful adventure called fatherhood. Throughout this book, I address uncertainties you may have, by giving you a weekly play-by-play. You'll find that you don't have to wait until the baby is born to get involved or until your child graduates from high school to truly start earning that Dad of the Year plaque, mug, or T-shirt.

Weekly Milestones

Each week opens with a quick glance at week-specific milestones. It's not unlike looking at your calendar on Monday morning to see what's ahead. Using insight and lessons from my own personal experiences with four pregnancies, each week begins with milestone openers that include vital pregnancy information—development stats on baby, Mom stats and what she's going through, and reminders and details about upcoming doctor's appointments or special events—that will tell you what you need to accomplish. Also, because not every week will have an important appointment or event or even a baby (Welcome to Week 1. Confusing, I know.), you get stats only when it's relevant so you can stay focused on what's in front of you.

Family Goals

It's not our responsibility to be mind readers when it comes to our partners' needs, but when it comes to pregnancy, we dads-to-be are just as accountable as our pregnant partners to be informed and own up to our part of the equation. To make it easier, I've structured the goals around the week-specific milestones so you're not left wondering what's happening, what's going to happen, or what you should be doing. If at the start and end of the day, all you did was just ask her vague questions about what you could do to help, you basically put all the onus back on her and rendered yourself useless. Be proactive and step up. Take ownership and prove to her, and most importantly to yourself, that you have the insight, confidence, and drive to have her back.

Just to be clear, when I talk about these weekly goals, I don't mean simply picking up takeout here and there when you happen to notice that she's too tired to cook, or taking out the trash before she has a chance to dispense the first reminder. To effectively relieve the stressors in her life while she is growing a human, especially because you can't offer to carry the baby for her, pull your weight by taking on the majority of the household chores. Make it your responsibility to load the dishwasher every night, tidy up the home, or prepare weekly meals. These are the kinds of practical, everyday goals that I'll be suggesting.

I also include goals that will help you start thinking ahead to the future—big-picture stuff. These types of goals include things such as making lists of questions to ask at the next doctor's appointment, considering a move if it's in your family's best interest, saving money to hire extra help if you need it, or talking to a financial adviser to gain perspective on budgeting or investing any extra money. These actions will help build sturdy bridges as you embark on your journey to growing a family.

While these day-to-day goals are meant to make a big impact, it's not always massive landmark decisions or things that need to be addressed—there are plenty of small moments and seemingly minor things that you might be inclined to do for your partner to help her relax, relieve some stress, or simply inspire a smile at an unexpected time.

Finally, while I did my best to cherry-pick simple day-to-day goals that resonate with most expectant partners and families, it's important to discuss your thought plan with your partner. Make sure that you are working toward the same goals, and always remember that communication is key. You might as well get used to falling back to that default and finding strength in it, since it will serve you well in pregnancy, parenthood, your partner relationship, and beyond.

Types of Goals and Support

Another reason I initially struggled with my wife's first pregnancy is because I didn't know what it meant to support her. Because this notion can be so vague and varied, I've categorized the family goals by the type of support you can offer during a particular week. You'll notice that certain kinds of support outnumber others, which clearly answers the *what* when asking about her needs and the things you can do. Here's the list of the types of support you'll encounter in this book. Feel free to add on to and personalize this list as you embark on this journey with your partner.

DAD RD *RD* stands for registered dietitian, so these goals have to do with keeping track of your partner's prenatal nutrition and making sure she is eating healthy by preparing foods that help with everything from morning sickness and fatigue to milk production and iron deficiency.

DADDY DOULA These goals involve anything that has to do with prenatal care (minus nutrition, as mentioned previously), labor, and postpartum care (namely breastfeeding) for Mom and baby.

HOME CEO These goals focus on taking on the majority of the chores or being proactive about what needs to be done around the house so that your partner doesn't have to worry about folding the laundry when her belly is swelling or answering vague questions about where stuff goes when she can't even see past that belly to her toes.

CONVERSATION STARTERS These are meant to spark discussion so you can address issues or things that could be potential issues later. These conversation starters are also meant to ensure that you keep communication constant and open.

BUDGET SAVVY Having a baby can be very expensive, so these goals help you establish and/or stick to a budget that fits your needs and lifestyle.

STRESS REDUCER Having a baby can also ramp up the anxiety meter, so these goals help your partner find physical and emotional relief when she needs it, or help you and your partner establish fun, comedic, and relaxing breaks so you can take a breather and refocus.

BONDING TIME It's easy to lose the intimacy in your relationship when you're having a baby, because your priorities inevitably change in the process. While some things won't be the same now that it's not just the two of you, there are still small things you can do to stay connected. These goals help you plan things like special dinners or dates and even bonding while preparing for baby.

FUN PROJECTS One of the best things about expecting is sharing your joy and happiness with family and friends—the people who matter the most—when the time is right. These goals help you plan things like baby announcements and gender reveals, which have become more sophisticated, easy, and interactive due to the latest upgrades in handheld devices, digital media, and social media.

PREGNANCY EMPATHY 101 It's hard to understand exactly what your pregnant partner is going through when you don't have the physiological requirements to have a baby yourself. That's why practicing empathy can take you far. These goals help put you in her shoes so you can better address her physical and emotional needs.

POSTPARTUM EMPATHY 101 This is the same goal as pregnancy empathy, but for the postpartum period, which is a time of painful recovery and continuing fluctuation of hormones that cause imbalanced moods and fatigue, all while learning how to breastfeed, soothe baby, and put baby to sleep. There's a lot that Mom is shouldering, and these goals help ensure that you understand what she needs during this challenging time.

PLAN AHEAD To ensure the best results or to prepare for the unexpected, planning ahead is key. These goals ensure that you are one step ahead, whether it's something as big as assessing your living situation before baby arrives or something smaller yet still impactful, like packing the hospital bag and creating a list of questions for the first baby appointment.

DADDY DAYCARE These suggestions have to do with baby duties, most often done solo, such as changing diapers, soothing baby, putting baby down to sleep, and playing with baby.

BROWNIE POINTS These goals are thoughtful things you can do to show your partner that you care about her well-being and appreciate all the work and sacrifices she is making to bring your baby into this world.

What Matters to Your Partner Should Matter to You, Too

You may still be wondering why you need to be so involved, especially since she already has her doctor, her books, her mom, her mom friends, and her instincts. You're probably also wondering when you'll have time to meet your own needs while you are busy with household chores and making lists of questions for the baby doctor. If you are still unsure about your role, I implore you to read on and learn.

During our first pregnancy, I'll never forget what my wife told me, "Women become mothers the moment they find out they're pregnant, and most men become fathers when they first hold their babies for the first time—but there are nine months in between." The reality is that it doesn't need to be this way and that we men should take ownership from the beginning. We need to make an effort to understand and realize that this isn't a solo journey. It all boils down to this simple realization: **What matters to your partner should matter to you because you're building a family**. In other words, it's no longer just about you, and whatever you do or don't do will have an impact on the whole family. Trust me on this.

The "Fourth Trimester"

The more involved a father is within the entire nine months of pregnancy, the more likely it is that he'll be ready for doing his part during those vital first three postpartum months, which many have come to know as the "fourth trimester." This term was coined from the notion that newborns are practically fetuses outside the womb for the first three months after they are born—they need to be constantly fed (every two hours or fed on demand) and kept neither too warm nor cold since newborns' bodies aren't equipped yet to regulate temperatures. The postpartum period requires a lot of mom and baby skin-to-skin bonding so that her body can increase milk production (if she wants to breastfeed) and keep baby warm and comforted.

What this all boils down to is that Mom *really* needs you in the trenches with her. She's recovering from the birth process or C-section as well as potentially breastfeeding around the clock and dealing with hormones that are in the beginning phase of regulating back to normal. Between recovery, sleep deprivation, and basic survival, these few weeks aren't easy on either parent.

Getting in on the ground floor and setting up the mentality that you're in this together will only make the "fourth trimester" less of a system shock for the both of you, and therefore more manageable. The better prepared both of you are, the better the family's overall well-being.

Once you're out of the hospital and settled at home, finding that routine or schedule with your partner is of paramount importance. A routine will relieve stress in both of your lives and allow you to put more emphasis on becoming great parents.

As a close friend of mine always says, "Fatherhood is the new brotherhood." Welcome to the club, Dad. You're gonna do great.

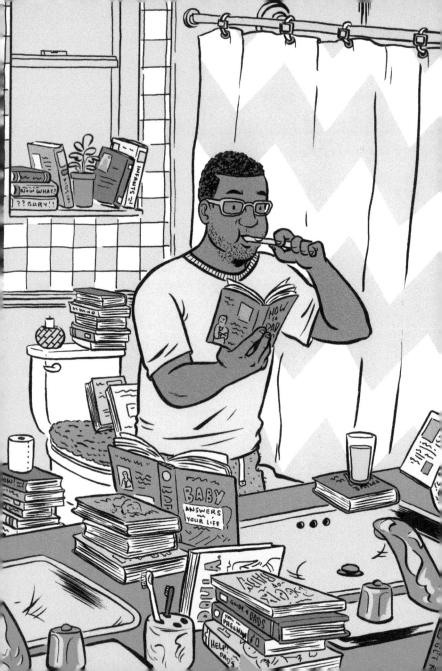

PART ONE

THE FIRST TRIMESTER

The first three months of pregnancy are some of the toughest, but I'm here to help! Whether you were planning your pregnancy or not, this adventure starts with a missed period. Don't spare any expense in investing in a reputable home pregnancy test to determine if this is the real deal. Once you and your partner have determined that she's pregnant, there will be a lot of questions about what to expect during the first several weeks. Part 1 of the book will answer those questions. You have been warned: We are going to refer to vocabulary like tender breasts and nipples, darkening or bumpy areolas, spotting, fatigue, bloating, and urinary frequency. Don't worry, they will most likely become everyday-speak before you know it. You'll eventually become an expert!

One of the most important things to consider about the first trimester is your current lifestyle. Things like booze and tobacco aren't conducive to fostering a healthy pregnancy. Mom should be adjusting her lifestyle with the idea that everything she puts in her body can and will have a direct effect on the baby. Eating healthy and getting enough rest are of paramount importance, and you can gently encourage this with your partner.

One of the first things you can do together as a couple is to research doctors (OB/GYNs, which stands for obstetrics and gynecology; obstetricians focus on pregnancy and childbirth, and gynecologists focus on overall female reproductive system health) in your area. If your partner doesn't already have an OB/GYN, get referrals from your primary care physician or crowdsource recommendations from friends and parents in your area. As you prepare for your initial appointment, knowing family history and important dates such as when your partner had her last period is key information to have available.

Keep in mind that over the next 12 weeks, Mom's body is preparing to carry a baby for the long haul, and with that comes intense hormonal changes. This is all normal, and Mom can use your support, whether it's physically or emotionally. As her partner, you're sort of silently tasked with making sure that she's doing okay with those changes and not overly affected with a prenatal mood disorder. Be there for her to help her relax or deal with any difficult issues.

Finding out that you're expecting, seeing your baby for the first time on an ultrasound, and potentially hearing the heartbeat are incredibly powerful and emotional moments in your life. Enjoy this amazing and intense bonding experience with your partner. Bringing a baby into this world isn't always easy. But it's a miracle and a blessing that should be treated as such.

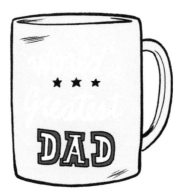

CHAPTER ONE

The First Month

If your partner has just become pregnant, you won't notice much in the way of physical or emotional changes just yet. There could be a touch of fatigue or tenderness in the breasts, but for the most part, Mom's body is preparing for the next eight months of growing another human. Sounds like a piece of cake, right? Wrong.

Now is the time for you and your partner to look at your lifestyle and consider whether it's conducive to bringing a beautiful baby into this world. Perhaps it's time to make some changes (or if you're fortunate, not many at all) as you become a father! Save those Bitcoins as an investment instead of spending them on questionable items online.

Although this pregnancy may not have a ton of impact on your life this month, it's never too early to be the best partner you can be and to provide support for Mom the rest of the way. Don't get stressed out; this is one of the most incredible adventures you'll experience in your life!

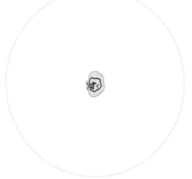

1-MONTH EMBRYO

NEW GEAR

placenta, umbilical cord, amniotic sac, tail

SIZE COMPARISON

poppy seed, grain of salt,
the period at the end of a sentence

Preparing for Pregnancy

One of the things that always confused me while attempting to track the course of my wife's pregnancy was the fact that there is no baby during Week 1. This is due to the fun fact that the first of the 40 weeks starts with the first day of your partner's last period. There's a reason for this—it's easier to track periods than ovulation, the signs of which aren't as noticeable in many women. This is also a reliable, internationally accepted standard for tracking pregnancy.

Over the years, my wife and I would jokingly refer to this time as "dating" or "practicing" to have a baby. With the first three pregnancies, we were fortunate enough (depending on how you look at it) to enjoy only one or two "dates" before the home pregnancy magic stick revealed the exciting news. I was ready for more practice!

Beginning with the latter part of my wife's third pregnancy, she was technically considered high risk because she was 35 years old, and it took more than a few "dates" to get pregnant—in actuality, it took months of us tracking her ovulation schedule and timing it just right to achieve the desired result. Note that even for the first few weeks of the 40 weeks, your partner won't experience any pregnancy symptoms or fetal

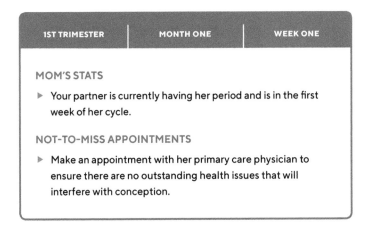

MOM'S STATS

▶ Your partner is currently having her period and is in the first week of her cycle.

NOT-TO-MISS APPOINTMENTS

▶ Make an appointment with her primary care physician to ensure there are no outstanding health issues that will interfere with conception.

growth, but she will be releasing an egg and setting the conditions for conception to occur. The stadium is getting set up for *the big game*.

Family Goals

PREGNANCY EMPATHY 101 Show an interest from the beginning: Since you're both committed to the idea of getting pregnant and starting a family, don't hesitate to talk openly about your expectations and fears. Conversely, ask your partner how she's feeling. There's absolutely nothing wrong with getting in on the ground floor and showing excitement for the possibility of bringing a beautiful baby into this world!

DAD RD Think like a dietitian: Your partner is likely taking prenatal vitamins loaded with folic acid, a pregnancy super vitamin that helps reduce the risk of neural tube (brain and spinal cord) defects. Folic acid is also found in foods like dried beans, peas, nuts, avocados, broccoli, collard greens, turnip greens, and okra. Unleash your inner chef and make something easy and delicious for her, like avocado toast. Or if you have time, turn on the slow cooker and crank out some pea soup. She and your future baby will thank you!

DADDY DOULA Encourage a healthy lifestyle: The party's over, Wayne! Remind her how important it is to avoid things like smoking and booze! Hopefully, she's way ahead of this reminder. And if you smoke or drink, maybe this is an opportunity to be selfless and go on hiatus or, at the very least, cut back while you're around her.

PREGNANCY EMPATHY 101 Be supportive while you're trying: Not everyone is able to get pregnant right away. Help your partner stay full of optimism to quash any unnecessary worry.

Ovulation and Fertilization

Day 14 of your partner's ovulation cycle is here. Wait, you didn't get the e-mail? That notification didn't pop up on your phone this morning? Maybe it won't always be this day, but it generally falls between days 12 and 16, so it's time to get busy.

This is the day that I referred to earlier as "dating" or "practicing." I'll be the first to admit, there is a lot of unnecessary pressure in the air on this one. Once the egg is released, it survives for about 12 to 24 hours, and it's then that fertilization will occur. The two of you should try to get on the same page about achieving the same goal here—to lead the healthiest lifestyle you can right now so all the energy and effort you put forward now will pay huge dividends in the end.

I don't personally know anyone who has actually used Barry White to set the mood, but it's time to get inspired. Go and crank up the jazz or that slow jams playlist you've been working on, drag a razor across your face, slap on the Acqua Di Giò, and find a shirt with a collar. It's magic hour (or several minutes in my case).

If fertilization of the egg occurs during this week, your baby is a zygote that has moved into the HOV lane of the fallopian tubes, headed toward the uterus. Even with the highest-performing

BABY'S STATS

▶ The ovum is meeting sperm.

▶ The egg may be fertilized this week, but it's tiny and could fit on the head of a pin.

MOM'S STATS

▶ Mom's period is over, and it's ovulation time.

▶ Her cervix may have increased mucus secretion, and she could potentially experience *mittelschmerz*, which is *not* a drinking game I invented in college. This is pain associated with the release of the egg, and most women won't even notice it.

▶ Estrogen levels are on the rise, and your partner may see a typical menstrual cycle weight gain of a half pound or so. On the flip side, she may also be more easily aroused as her body pushes toward fertilization, so cue the 1970s porn music.

NOT-TO-MISS APPOINTMENTS

▶ Sexy time on your partner's ovulation cycle.

sperm specimen, it will still take the sperm between three and five days to get to the uterus for implantation.

A simple way for you to keep your secret calendar straight is to remember 7, 14, 21, and 28. If your partner has a typical

28-day cycle, her period is the first week, day 14 is ovulation, day 21 is implantation, and day 28 is when the needle on the record goes all the way back to the beginning.

Family Goals

DADDY DOULA Let Mom get some rest: Sleep is of the utmost importance. There's no harm in Mom beginning to get into a pattern of healthy sleep while trying to get pregnant. Be respectful of your shared space—no need to keep her up till midnight with Cris Collinsworth's lackadaisical *Sunday Night Football* commentary blaring on the other side of the wall.

DAD RD Keep focusing on nutrition: Nutrition will continue to be of paramount importance for the next nine months, and beyond if Mom is breastfeeding. Think about surprising your partner with a nice Moleskine journal and encourage her to keep track of what she's eating and how much physical activity she logs during the week. Maybe even knock out an agreement to exercise together—it could be a nice change of pace to take a walk together after work.

BROWNIE POINTS Wine and dine, or just dine: Who says trying for a baby has to be work? Before getting busy, treat the night as an actual date. Ask her out to dinner and a movie. Who knows, maybe you'll have so much fun that you'll forget you're trying, and stress-free baby-making is exactly what her body needs.

Conception

If everything has worked out the way it was supposed to, your sperm has built up speed, caught some magnificent air, and landed directly inside of the egg, à la the high-tech assault vehicle in *Tango & Cash*. This point of contact creates the zygote. The zygote has finished its journey through the fallopian tubes and is continuing its cell division and multiplication. I know, I know. Sit down, take an Advil, and rub some essential oils on your temples—math was never my thing either.

The fertilized cell (zygote) divides for the first time within hours of the sperm meeting the egg. It continues to divide, and within several days, it has matured into a ball of cells—which, to put things into perspective, is significantly smaller than the period that concludes this sentence.

Congratulations, you've now got a blastocyst! This term may not be the cutest nickname to give your growing baby, and I'm guessing that you and your partner may eventually come up with something a little more fitting. In our family and extended family, it's been called everything from pea to bean to sprout, and Skittle to jelly bean to gumdrop. You may prefer something with a little more machismo, for instance, Rambo or the Enforcer or Lil' Charles Bronson. Totally your call.

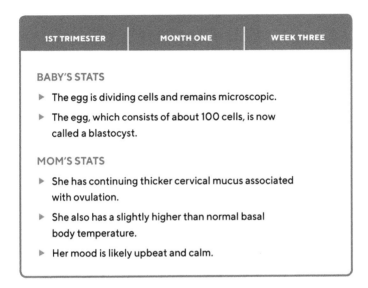

BABY'S STATS

▶ The egg is dividing cells and remains microscopic.

▶ The egg, which consists of about 100 cells, is now called a blastocyst.

MOM'S STATS

▶ She has continuing thicker cervical mucus associated with ovulation.

▶ She also has a slightly higher than normal basal body temperature.

▶ Her mood is likely upbeat and calm.

Family Goals

BROWNIE POINTS Leave room for dessert: Mom may notice a slight increase in appetite this week with the building hormonal changes. No need to criticize the volume of food intake—in fact, if you're making dinner at home, it might be nice to pick up a surprise treat. And, no, pickles and ice cream probably isn't your best bet.

Implantation and the Great Divide

This is an exciting yet nerve-racking week for you and Mom. Once she realizes that she's missed her period, she's in the clear to take a home pregnancy test, although the accuracy won't reach its peak until about one week after the missed period. It can be a really difficult thing to wait for the right day to take a pregnancy test. You *can* get a false negative if she tests too early; however, it's nearly impossible to get a false positive.

Home pregnancy tests check for the hCG hormone, which begins to increase exponentially following implantation. Some pregnancy tests can tell you the results several days before your partner's missed period (typically on day 28), but unless you buy one of these tests, you are better off waiting, to ward off unnecessary disappointment.

Your little ball of cells is now officially called an embryo. It has reached the uterus and is nestling into the uterine lining, where it will take up permanent residence and stay connected until delivery. It's here and now that the embryo begins what is referred to as the "great divide": It splits into two groups. One of these groups will become your son or daughter and the other

BABY'S STATS

▶ The ball of cells continues to increase in size and is now about the size of a poppy seed.

▶ Your baby is now officially considered an embryo.

▶ Baby's organs begin to develop this week!

MOM'S STATS

▶ The embryo is attaching itself to the uterine lining, a process referred to as "implantation."

▶ Some women may notice implantation with slight bleeding and cramping about 7 to 12 days after ovulation. This will likely occur as spotting, accompanied by what feels like period cramps.

▶ Mom may also notice some breast changes this week, such as increased nipple sensitivity, soreness, tenderness, or swelling.

▶ An increase in urination is generally one of pregnancy's earliest signs.

NOT-TO-MISS APPOINTMENTS

▶ If the home pregnancy test yields a positive result, you need to schedule an appointment right away with your OB/GYN or midwife.

will become the placenta, your baby's lifeline during his or her uterine stay.

The amniotic sac—also referred to as the bag of waters—is beginning to form, as is the yolk sac that will eventually become incorporated into your baby's developing digestive tract. Each layer of the embryo (a total of three now) is beginning to grow into specialized parts of the body.

▶ Endoderm—the inner layer that eventually becomes the digestive system, liver, and lungs

▶ Mesoderm—the middle layer that eventually becomes the baby's heart, sex organs, bones, kidneys, and muscles

▶ Ectoderm—the outer layer that eventually becomes the nervous system, hair, skin, and eyes

See how much is happening? Why wasn't I taking it upon myself to be a supportive partner the first time around? Hindsight is always 20/20, and perhaps I'm in a much different place now that I'm older and more mature, but I now find this process so incredibly fascinating.

Family Goals

 CONVERSATION STARTERS Reassess your living situation:

Where are you living? Is it a healthy environment in which to raise a baby? These are questions that you and your partner should

ask yourselves when you are having a frank discussion about whether moving is in your future. If you don't think you have enough space for a new addition to the family, be proactive and start using some basic services like Zillow, Trulia, or Apartment Guide to dial in on a fresh new start. If not, maybe you can find ways to improve the condition of your current residence.

Do you have enough space for a nursery? My wife and I lived in a two-bedroom apartment in West Los Angeles when we found out that she was pregnant. While apprehensive at first, I had to convert that second bedroom (my home office/man cave) into the nursery, complete with pink accent walls and chiffon curtains.

What life changes need to be made to ensure that you're ready to welcome a baby home in 8½ months? The reality is that poker night may have to be moved to a different location—no groups of eight guys smoking cigars and crushing half-gallons of Captain Morgan in your living room while Mom is trying to rest.

DADDY DOULA Plan to spot her during upcoming prenatal appointments: Communicate with your partner and insist on going with her once the first prenatal visit is scheduled—the experience of easing the stress *and* holding hands in the waiting room is a memory and feeling that you'll never forget.

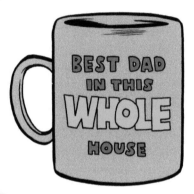

CHAPTER TWO

The Second Month

On the surface, Mom's body still isn't showing much in the way of being pregnant, and chances are that you and your partner have chosen not to mention anything to anyone yet. But just because you can't tell that she's growing a baby doesn't mean that she isn't feeling it.

Mom is growing more fatigued by the day. Her nausea is increasing, and she may be starting to experience morning sickness. There are massive hormonal changes happening within her body, and her breasts are preparing themselves to produce milk. Her nipples are incredibly sore, so watch the funny business!

Your partner is going to need every bit of your support— at this point, general encouragement about eating healthy, getting moderate exercise, and treating her body like a temple. You'll want to help her create a perfect environment inside of her body but also do your part in making her home life serene.

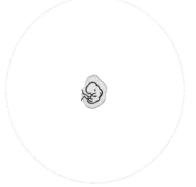

2-MONTH FETUS

NEW GEAR

face, eye, hand, foot, neural tube, heart

SIZE COMPARISON

raspberry, jelly bean, Aspirin pill

The Neural Tube

I've always felt like that first month of pregnancy came and went before I even had a chance to acknowledge what was happening with my wife. Even though your partner might not be showing, so much is going on.

The embryo is beginning to look less and less like a ball of cells and more like a tadpole. Remember last week when we talked about that outer layer of cells called the ectoderm? This is where the neural tube is developing, which will be the building block for the entire nervous system and spine.

The middle layer, the mesoderm, is where the circulatory system, skeleton, and very early beginnings of the heart and vessels are developing. The third layer, the endoderm, will eventually contain your baby's organs, but for now it connects to the placenta, which is transporting all the necessary nutrients to help it grow.

On the outside, Mom probably doesn't look much different; however, she will tend to notice occasional nausea, breast tenderness, and an increasing urge to urinate as she moves forward.

BABY'S STATS

▶ Your baby is the size of a small lemon seed.

▶ The heart, which is about the size of a poppy seed, is starting to take shape and beginning to beat.

▶ The neural tube is open but will close next week. This will eventually become the brain and spinal cord.

MOM'S STATS

▶ She has continuing breast tenderness and possible enlargement.

▶ She has continuing frequent urination.

▶ She may have nausea.

▶ Her fatigue begins to show.

NOT-TO-MISS APPOINTMENTS

▶ You've hopefully already scheduled the first appointment with your doctor or midwife.

Family Goals

HOME CEO Be in charge of the main household chores: Try to look at it this way . . . Whether Mom currently works full time out of the home or not, she's just inherited a second job—growing a human inside her. Look around the house and evaluate the top things that need to be done to maintain a sane household. This especially applies to the situation where Mom-to-be usually delegates what goes on around the house, especially the cleaning. The fatigue that Mom's feeling is legit. Offer to do her share of the household chores, and encourage her to relax and kick her feet up for a bit. Perhaps it might help to "learn the system" that's in place *or* suggest that you reorganize some things around the house to fit with what works best for you. Side note: Most women find it sexy watching their man tidy up the place.

DADDY DOULA Alert Mom when you're out and about and bathrooms become available: You'll be surprised at how frequently she will have to urinate. Be a sport and remind her to go before you get in the car, and be patient if she needs to stop en route and go again. And again.

Your Baby Has a Face

I always found it funny when books or online resources would tell me that "my baby has a face." I'd instantly picture a little Chris Farley, Jack Nicholson, or Oprah.

The reality is that your baby isn't telling you that he lives in a van down by the river, donning a velvet Los Angeles Lakers tracksuit and Ray-Bans, or hosting a daytime talk show. It's still only the size of a Skittle, and while the head is a big portion of the crown-to-rump measurement (a quarter inch or so), the eyes, ears, and nose are just beginning to form and become more distinct. That little beating heart is pumping blood through its tiny vessels, and the little nubs that will eventually be the arms and legs are beginning to be noticeable.

Mom still isn't showing much in the waist, but her nipples are darkening, and her breasts are getting larger. Her hair may be getting thicker as hormones keep it from falling out, *and* her nails may also be getting stronger and longer.

BABY'S STATS

▶ The fetus is developing eyes, ears, a jaw, cheeks, and a chin.

▶ The kidneys, liver, and lungs are taking shape.

▶ The heart is beating 110 times per minute.

MOM'S STATS

▶ Mom is too small to show yet, but she may have a certain "glow" about her.

▶ Her hair may be thicker and her nails may be stronger.

▶ She has larger breasts and darker nipples.

▶ Her hormones could be causing mood swings.

NOT-TO-MISS APPOINTMENTS

▶ Week 6 is the most common week for your first prenatal appointment. Urine and blood will be screened for nutrient deficiencies, and Mom will be weighed and have her blood pressure tested.

▶ The doctor may also do a very quick pelvic exam.

Family Goals

CONVERSATION STARTERS Prepare for the first prenatal appointment: Ask your partner if she's come up with a list of questions to ask her doctor. And one *important note*: You should also be prepared with knowing the first and last day of Mom's last period. She'll be surprised that you were paying attention.

DADDY DOULA Encourage exercise: Okay, maybe you don't need to channel your inner Mr. Miyagi, and it's probably not appropriate to ask your partner to sand fences or practice the crane kick, but encouraging some daily exercise is great for her and for the baby's health. Remember those his 'n' hers Fitbits you bought for Valentine's Day? Time to break them out.

DADDY DOULA Be on the lookout for prenatal mood disorders: Being aware of the potential for anxiety and depression is the best way to manage this concern. Keep in mind that a majority of women hold these feelings in, so you might have to get inquisitive with your partner and ask some questions.

QUESTIONS FOR THE FIRST PRENATAL APPOINTMENT

▶ *How much weight should she be gaining and at what rate?*

▶ *Given her age, should she be concerned about any specific conditions or restrictions?*

▶ *Does she need any specific screenings, and if so when will they occur?*

▶ *What about diet? Are there certain foods she should eat? What should she stay away from?*

▶ *Is she allowed to exercise? For how long?*

▶ *Can my partner continue having sex? Are there any restrictions?*

▶ *Can she travel without restriction? For how long?*

▶ *Can she dye her hair? Get massages?*

▶ *Should she be taking prenatal vitamins?*

▶ *What if she has additional questions? When can she call or e-mail you?*

Hands and Feet

This week is full of signals—some that might be crossed and others that might be right on the money. The baby is growing at an outrageous rate, and its skeleton has fully formed. The skeleton is not the hard bone that we're accustomed to seeing but rather is soft and pliable. Those nubs that we talked about last week are now looking more paddle-like and dividing into hand, arm, and shoulder segments, along with leg, knee, and foot segments. The baby's digestive system, kidneys, liver, pancreas, and appendix are now developed. Thankfully, you won't have to worry about changing those stinky diapers for another few months.

Mom is probably beginning to feel a little rough around the edges. The nausea, morning sickness, and/or aversion to certain foods may have dramatically increased. This time in the pregnancy is one that has stuck in my head each time we've been fortunate enough to have another child on the way. It feels like with almost every pregnancy, like clockwork, one day my wife would wake up and begin sniffing around the house, her nose scrunched up into her eye sockets. The *super smell* had arrived.

First, she would focus on my gym shoes or our daughter's UGGs that she wears for weeks without socks. Then she'd move on to my truck or our son's bedroom closet (where the dog buried

BABY'S STATS

▶ Your baby is as big as a blueberry and 10,000 times bigger than at conception!

▶ The entire skeleton has formed, yet it's still soft and pliable.

▶ The brain is developing at a rate of 100 cells per minute.

▶ The digestive system, kidneys, liver, appendix, and pancreas are helping with waste management.

▶ The nubs that will eventually form the arms and legs are continuing to grow and will soon divide into hands and feet.

MOM'S STATS

▶ Her uterus has doubled in size to accommodate the baby.

▶ The placenta has now developed hairlike projections called "villi" that are transferring nutrients from Mom to baby.

▶ She might have morning sickness and/or food aversions.

▶ A sixth sense emerges: *super smell.*

▶ Pregnancy cravings may start.

NOT-TO-MISS APPOINTMENTS

▶ If you had your appointment during Week 6, then you were probably told by your doctor that you should discuss completing prenatal testing for genetic or chromosomal conditions.

a half slice of pizza months earlier that had turned into a science experiment). Eventually, her super smell inevitably led her to the kitchen refrigerator and, without warning, I had a new skill set to add to my LinkedIn résumé: I was officially promoted to the "guy in charge of smelling things to see if they're rotten."

What did that mean? If there was anything in the refrigerator that could be potentially close to its expiration date, I would be designated to stick my nose in it to figure out where we stood.

My wife didn't stand a chance when it came to sour cream, old milk, blue cheese, or "fermented" ravioli that I'd somehow forgotten to throw out. For her, it would mean *hurl city*.

Family Goals

HOME CEO Freshen up the house: That super smell is no joke. Think about doing some deep cleaning around the house. Rent or buy a steam cleaner for the carpets. Scrub out that refrigerator and freezer and get rid of stuff that has seen better days. Drag those various trash cans into the front yard like Cousin Eddie (of *National Lampoon's Christmas Vacation*) would, hose them out with a little soap, and you're back in business.

DAD RD Expand your cooking repertoire: Find different ways to cook produce—try roasting root vegetables like beets or baby carrots, maybe even Brussels sprouts or cauliflower.

BONDING TIME Dine alfresco: If it's nice outside, research some regional or state parks in your area. Chances are they have some easy trails that you could take on. If you want to combine both ideas, roll up a blanket and pack some sparkling water, a hard cheese (soft cheese isn't good for pregnant women), and some crackers, and you've got yourself a date.

BROWNIE POINTS Surround her with her favorite fragrances: If you really want to live on the wild side, find out what smells *she does like*. Then be sure to swing by T.J. Maxx on your way home from work and grab a lilac or sandalwood diffuser like a real man!

Fingers and Toes

You can breathe easy this week, as your baby's tail is almost gone. Go have a cold one and hit the showers!

Just kidding. There's a bunch more going on that you need to catch up on . . .

Congratulations are in order not only because your baby is looking less reptilian and more human but also because it now has eyelids and is developing lungs. Its tiny heart is beating *twice* as fast as yours, and the baby is beginning to make spontaneous twitching movements. Fingers and toes are beginning to show more definition. However, the digits do still resemble those of a frog or "that guy" at the community pool who uses webbed swim gear and paddles laps around you like he's training for the Summer Olympics.

Toes can be an interesting thing to stress about. Will he or she have regular toes like the author's or Morton's toe (the second toe is longer than the big toe) like my wife's? It's an ongoing, intense debate in our home.

Either way, toes are toes, and they're beautiful. He or she just may have to be careful when choosing flip-flops or open-toed shoes for special engagements. For years, my wife contended that a Morton's toe meant that you were smarter

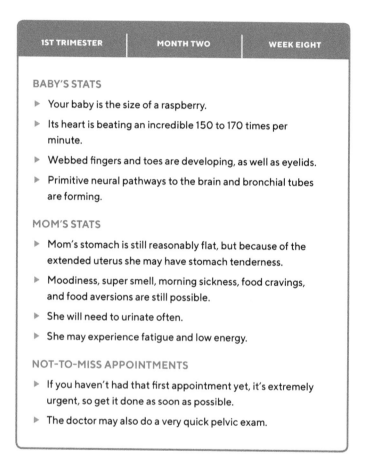

BABY'S STATS

► Your baby is the size of a raspberry.

► Its heart is beating an incredible 150 to 170 times per minute.

► Webbed fingers and toes are developing, as well as eyelids.

► Primitive neural pathways to the brain and bronchial tubes are forming.

MOM'S STATS

► Mom's stomach is still reasonably flat, but because of the extended uterus she may have stomach tenderness.

► Moodiness, super smell, morning sickness, food cravings, and food aversions are still possible.

► She will need to urinate often.

► She may experience fatigue and low energy.

NOT-TO-MISS APPOINTMENTS

► If you haven't had that first appointment yet, it's extremely urgent, so get it done as soon as possible.

► The doctor may also do a very quick pelvic exam.

and more creative; however, upon further research, I was able to say: "According to Google, you're totally wrong!" (which felt fantastic, but I digress).

Family Goals

STRESS REDUCER Find a fun diversion to relieve stress: Mom's pregnancy hormones are definitely kicking in. Finding a fun distraction for her mood swings and anxiety is a good thing. What can you do to keep her mind off things? Invite friends over to play Cards Against Humanity? Challenge her to a game of Scrabble? What about a game of mini-golf?

PREGNANCY EMPATHY 101 Listen more, talk less: Mom's hormones are brewing as her body prepares itself for the next several months, which may cause some abrupt shifts in mood. Be patient and hear her out, even if it sometimes feels as if the conversation isn't as relevant as it normally might be.

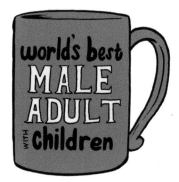

CHAPTER THREE

The Third Month

This month is a huge milestone in the pregnancy. Your partner is coming up to the end of the first trimester. Even though her fatigue is ramping up and she's finding herself going to the bathroom several more times during the day than usual, there is light at the end of the tunnel.

If she's experiencing morning sickness, the end is in sight (if she's like most women). But that doesn't change the fact that her uterus is continuously expanding, and as her belly grows, mild discomfort and trouble sleeping are other factors that will begin to pop up.

But the exciting part about this month is that you'll most likely have your first doctor's appointment, *and* chances are good that you'll be able to hear your baby's heartbeat for the first time—which is a life-changing experience all on its own. The conclusion of this month also brings a drastic reduction in the potential for miscarriage, and it may also mean that you and your partner choose to tell those close to you the good news. It'll feel good to let family and friends in on your amazing secret!

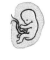

3-MONTH FETUS

NEW GEAR

mouth, nose, ears, arms, toes, fingers, bones,
organs: intestines, liver, kidney, bladder

SIZE COMPARISON

slightly bigger than a lime, toy soldier

Starting to Look Like a Person

Entering month 3, your baby is about one inch long, almost the same size as a martini olive. It'll still be another couple of months before Mom is able to feel the kicks and punches of your little one, but that doesn't mean that your baby isn't full of life. Its tiny heart has started beating!

There were certainly times between doctor's appointments when my wife felt nervous and simply wanted the comfort of hearing our baby's heartbeat when she got home from work or before she took a warm (not hot!) bath before bedtime.

As baby starts to develop, anxiety around life stats might ramp up. Do your best to keep things calm and find manageable solutions.

Family Goals

DAD RD Make a soothing tea from fresh ginger: Dad, it's time to get to know ginger. No, I'm not talking about the character from *Gilligan's Island* or the NFL's best quarterback, Carson Wentz of the Philadelphia Eagles, but rather the Chinese root that looks like gnarled fingers. This can be a huge weapon against the nausea associated with

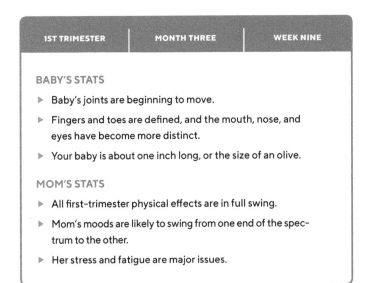

BABY'S STATS

▶ Baby's joints are beginning to move.

▶ Fingers and toes are defined, and the mouth, nose, and eyes have become more distinct.

▶ Your baby is about one inch long, or the size of an olive.

MOM'S STATS

▶ All first-trimester physical effects are in full swing.

▶ Mom's moods are likely to swing from one end of the spectrum to the other.

▶ Her stress and fatigue are major issues.

morning sickness. You can usually find it in the produce section of any decent grocery store. Use a vegetable peeler to take the skin off one of the nubs, shred it, boil it, and give it to Mom to drink as a tea with a little honey or sugar.

STRESS REDUCER Consider a Doppler: Ever since our first pregnancy, my wife and I have rented a device from a company called BabyBeat that allows you to hear your baby's heartbeat—a handheld Doppler. It will generally run you about $25 to $35 per month. If this is your first pregnancy and you plan to have more children, you may even consider buying one instead of renting; they're relatively inexpensive, and owning can be more cost effective in the long run. This portable device has been a lifesaver when it comes to relieving stress, letting go of the worry, and getting a good night's sleep. Don't get discouraged if it takes many, many tries to get zoned in on the heartbeat. With continued practice and the natural progression of the pregnancy, this becomes much easier, and you'll be a pro.

Finally a Fetus

Week 10 is one of those huge landmarks within the first trimester. This is the week that your embryo finally becomes a fetus. The elbows are beginning to work, little teeth buds are forming below the gum line, and if it's a boy, the testes are starting to develop. This might be the week that Mom begins to see some outward growth when it comes to the baby bump. If you had your first doctor's appointment on the early side, you should probably think about checking in with your doctor, as prenatal test results will be coming soon.

Family Goals

BUDGET SAVVY Set a budget for maternity clothes: As Mom begins to sport her new bump, it may be time to start saving for maternity clothes. Do a little online research first because maternity jeans aren't necessarily cheap. It might be a good week to switch back to domestics and give the craft beers a break to cover the spread. For those of you who are on your second or third pregnancy, it might be time to get your ass into the basement or attic to find that

BABY'S STATS

▶ Baby has officially graduated from embryo to fetus.

▶ All vital organs are in place.

▶ Baby's bones and cartilage are forming, along with knees and ankles.

▶ Baby has a bulging forehead with a growing brain, fingernails, and toenails.

MOM'S STATS

▶ Her uterus has doubled in size—from a pear to a grapefruit.

▶ This could be the week that the baby bump makes its appearance.

▶ A bigger bra and maternity clothes are in the future.

▶ She might experience ligament pain in the abdomen as it stretches to accommodate the baby.

▶ Her mood swings are still in effect.

NOT-TO-MISS APPOINTMENTS

▶ You'll most likely schedule your second appointment with the doctor and review the results of the initial prenatal testing. Typically, Mom's weight, blood pressure, and urine are also checked. Genetic blood testing (not necessarily covered by insurance unless she's high risk) could potentially occur during this appointment if you've decided to have it done.

▶ The nuchal translucency scan (NT scan) tests for Down syndrome or other chromosomal abnormalities.

30-gallon bin of clothes from the last go-round and crank up your washer and dryer for an all-out laundry campaign.

BONDING TIME Wind down with Mom: Even though our interests are different, my wife and I occasionally share mutual affection for a series on Netflix or network TV. We often try to have dinner on Sunday nights and binge-watch to catch up. Before we had kids, we would eat dinner in the bedroom, which was the perfect end to a stressful week and helped us reset for the tough week that lay ahead.

DADDY DOULA Suggest a yoga class: With Mom's ligament pains becoming more and more prevalent in her abdomen, a prenatal yoga class might be just what the daddy ordered.

BROWNIE POINTS Take her shopping: As Mom's uterus continues to grow, so will her belly. Those skinny jeans and tight tops aren't going to cut it anymore. Suggest a lunch date to go with her to try on some new stuff *or* encourage her to reach out to a close friend who was recently pregnant herself and borrow some gently used clothing stored away.

Teeth and Bones

There may not be a lot to notice when it comes to Mom's outward appearance this week. Despite the fact that the baby is probably less than the length of your thumb, Mom is beginning to gain a little bit of weight here and there. Week 11 was always an exciting time for my wife and me. We had already visited our doctor for the first prenatal visit and had the first ultrasound. We always followed the 12-week rule: We didn't tell anyone outside our immediate family that she was pregnant until we hit that third month. The percentage chance of miscarriage tends to drop significantly when the first trimester comes to a close. My wife and I experienced a miscarriage early in our first trimester in between babies three and four. It was truly a devastating time for us. The bittersweet layer that made it a little easier was knowing that so many of our friends had sadly been through similar experiences to ours; realizing we didn't "do anything wrong" was extremely healing to us. The biggest thing that was really important for us to take away from that loss was the idea of telling some people earlier than 12 weeks. It's important to tell people about your pregnancy early if they're the people you would call if a miscarriage were to occur and you needed their help or support. During our miscarriage,

BABY'S STATS

▶ Baby is about 1½ inches long, weighs about a quarter ounce, and its head is about half of its body size.

▶ Baby's bones are hardening, its torso is lengthening, and its hair follicles and fingernail and toenail beds are beginning to develop.

▶ Buds of teeth are forming under the gums.

▶ Baby's organs continue to develop and grow.

MOM'S STATS

▶ Mom may have a baby bump on display right now.

▶ Maternity clothes are beginning to make their debut.

▶ Mom has likely gained one to five pounds.

NOT-TO-MISS APPOINTMENTS

▶ Make sure that you've got that second prenatal appointment set.

we had to tell our parents not only that we were pregnant but also that we had miscarried at the same time, and it was a really horrible situation. Hindsight is 20/20, though, and we learned from that and decided to clue in those closest to us as soon as we got our first positive pregnancy test.

ON MISCARRIAGES

Given where we are in the time line of pregnancy, it bears mentioning that miscarriages are unfortunately a common occurrence. There are numerous factors that lead to miscarriages, including age (over 35), lifestyle, diet, chronic conditions, and medical emergencies such as an ectopic pregnancy. The loss of a child at any age or developmental stage is devastating, so if it does happen to you and your partner, stick together and be supportive of one another. And please *don't* let it affect you to the point that you stop trying. The Resources section (page 272) recommends some places where you can go for support and grief counseling.

Because you've now hit the 11-week mark, this is as good a time as any to start talking about how you're going to announce the fact that you're pregnant. Whether you're a first-timer or a repeat parent, this is an exciting time for you and everyone in your social circles. Social media (especially Facebook) has made it significantly easier to deliver big announcements like this in an easy, sweeping fashion. You'll be surprised how much stress is relieved, as well as how many old friends come out of the woodwork to share in your joy.

Family Goals

CONVERSATION STARTERS Discuss whom to tell among your core people: This is probably the most difficult week to keep your secret. Mom's belly is starting to pop out, and most couples try to wait until the end of the first trimester to begin announcing the great news to family, friends, and the dreaded Facebook. Discuss with your partner whom you think you should tell. I know that in our case, there were certain people we felt should know before they read about it on Twitter.

FUN PROJECTS Plan the reveal: Come up with creative ideas on how to tell your family and close friends. Maybe you have a good friend who is a photographer, or maybe you get a referral, but this is a great week to hire someone for an hour to do a baby bump photo shoot as a teaser photo for the announcement. The photos can also be used in your private photo album.

BUDGET SAVVY Buy jeans extenders: As her belly begins to grow, Mom-to-be will find it difficult to close her jeans button. She's outgrowing her normal clothes, but she's not exactly ready for maternity clothes. Before you blow the budget on things you are not quite sure she will really need when normal clothes are completely out of the question, buy her jeans extenders so she can still use her regular jeans while you both keep that maternity clothes budget intact. Bellabands are $25 bands that allow Mom to wear her pants unzipped with a band around the waist so she can get much more mileage out of them.

Reflexes

Your baby has *doubled* in size over the past few weeks, and the development process is in full effect. Baby has started to make sucking motions to prepare for eating and will most likely respond to external stimuli, but it is still way too small for Mom to be able to feel anything.

Your partner is getting really close to the end of the first trimester, and this pregnancy begins to feel real for both of you. Personally, I remember this time during every pregnancy that we've shared together. My wife's bump was beginning to show, she was buying new maternity jeans (or digging old ones out of the attic), and wearing flowy, loose shirts, and I was carrying an air of pride everywhere we went.

There was a certain element of protectiveness and sensitivity that began growing within me. I was going out of my way to open doors and help my wife into our truck—things that I should normally be doing, but for some reason this chivalrous feeling was reinvigorated within me. Hang on. For most guys, this is where the journey really feels like it's taking off!

BABY'S STATS

▶ Your baby is the size of a lime.

▶ Baby's intestines, eyes, and ears are in place.

▶ Baby begins getting reflexes, although it is still too small for Mom to notice movements.

▶ Baby begins to respond to external stimuli.

MOM'S STATS

▶ The top of the uterus is above the pelvic bones.

▶ She has potential discomfort lying on her stomach, as her uterus presses on her abdomen.

▶ She has occasional indigestion.

▶ Mom's moodiness and serious fatigue may begin to wane.

NOT-TO-MISS APPOINTMENTS

▶ See Week 10 as a reminder to make that important second-trimester appointment.

Family Goals

FUN PROJECTS Plan your pregnancy announcement: If you talked last week about the PR strategy
for announcing your pregnancy, take it to the next level.
Research some photo templates or the best way to get your
finished product printed and shipped. We also FaceTimed
with parents, siblings, and extended family, and we delivered
the news in person or by e-mail over a weekend to her
employers. Once that was done, we felt comfortable putting
up a social media post that blanketed everyone else.

BONDING TIME Plan a trip: This is a superb time to
begin planning a trip together. Before long, it may be
too difficult for Mom to maneuver and instead of roasting
your yams walking around Colonial Williamsburg, she might
enjoy sitting poolside on a chaise lounge in Palm Springs.
Not that there's anything wrong with historical vacations;
it's just that relaxing is a whole lot better. Just make sure
that you don't plan any flights after Week 36. (I cover this
again later in the book.)

Call It a Trimester

While Mom's baby bump is only now beginning to become completely undeniable, there have been other changes that aren't so subtle. If you've been tuned in to your partner, she's gone through a fair number of physical changes that, for a new mom on her first pregnancy who isn't expecting them, can be a tough pill to swallow. Headaches are a frequent offender. The main reason for the influx of simple headaches or the more complex migraine headaches (I get these and don't wish them on even my worst enemy) is pregnancy hormones.

You're probably thinking, "Big deal. It's a headache. Take something and move on." But most of the normal remedies out there are off-limits and could potentially have negative effects on the fetus. And while she may not have shared her tribulations with you, constipation is another big issue as she closes out the first trimester. With her uterus expanding and growing another human, it tends to act like a belligerent drunk pushing his way to the bar to squeeze another drink in before Happy Hour officially ends.

The other changes Mom is experiencing are emotional. It's certainly not uncommon to all of a sudden think your partner has gone off the deep end. With all those raging hormones, her moods can swing like a pendulum—one minute, you're

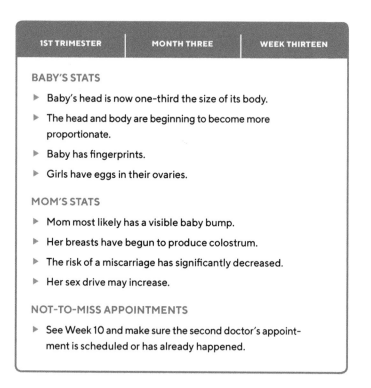

BABY'S STATS

▶ Baby's head is now one-third the size of its body.

▶ The head and body are beginning to become more proportionate.

▶ Baby has fingerprints.

▶ Girls have eggs in their ovaries.

MOM'S STATS

▶ Mom most likely has a visible baby bump.

▶ Her breasts have begun to produce colostrum.

▶ The risk of a miscarriage has significantly decreased.

▶ Her sex drive may increase.

NOT-TO-MISS APPOINTMENTS

▶ See Week 10 and make sure the second doctor's appointment is scheduled or has already happened.

the sweetest hubby who ever existed and the next, you're the shittiest person on the face of the earth for not putting the TV remote back where it belongs.

Family Goals

DAD RD Make smaller meals: The best ways to help her combat her constipation are to make smaller meals and to helpfully suggest that she doesn't gorge at mealtime. Consider breaking three squares down to five or six smaller meals throughout the day—grazing instead of trying to win a competitive eating competition. Also, *fluids*. Water and juice tend to soften stool, and with regular intake they should help alleviate having to set up a temporary office in the loo.

PREGNANCY EMPATHY 101 Support emotional changes: Be patient and understanding. After four pregnancies, I know this shift in emotions is coming and often go out of my way to keep things tidy and make it so there shouldn't be much that she can get upset about.

BONDING TIME Plan a date night: For many moms, as those pregnancy hormones rage, her sex drive increases. Between the hormones and newly formed curves and larger-than-life breasts, it's not uncommon for her to feel like the sexual thermostat has been cranked up. Perhaps now is a great time to plan a night out: Have dinner (no gorging—maybe try a tapas joint) and see a movie. Follow it up with giving her a foot rub at home and surprising her with her favorite frozen ice cream—then see where this whole thing goes . . .

DADDY DOULA Help her with the headaches: There are a few simple ways to avoid the headache altogether. Make sure your partner is eating regularly and reducing the stress in her life, and help her make time to find a quiet and calm place to relax. You'll be surprised at how these little things can go a long way.

THE FIRST-TRIMESTER CHECKLIST

HOME:

☐ Discuss your living situation with your partner. Focus on having your home ready for when the baby arrives.

☐ Assume control of the household. The goal is to have mom feel less stress and to take over the responsibility over running the household.

☐ Set a budget for maternity clothes.

☐ Start researching your bigger baby purchases like car seats, strollers, and video cameras.

☐ Make sure your insurance covers life, disability, homeowners or rental, auto, and any other special coverage you may need

BABY:

☐ Nutrition will be of the utmost importance. Although your baby isn't around yet, make sure mom is eating well and getting enough nutritious foods.

☐ Plan the announcement: figure out a fun way to announce your new baby to your loved ones.

MOM:

- ☐ Make sure she cuts smoking and alcohol, if it applies to her.
- ☐ Help her get onto a regular sleep cycle and a daily exercise regimen.
- ☐ Take her shopping for maternity clothes.
- ☐ Plan a trip: the second trimester is the ideal time to go on a trip before it becomes too difficult for her to travel, so start planning now.

PRENATAL APPOINTMENTS:

- ☐ Between four to eight weeks is the first visit for the following:
    - ☐ Blood test
    - ☐ Ultrasound (for heartbeat)
    - ☐ Physical exam
    - ☐ Pelvic exam
    - ☐ Overview of prenatal care for the next eight months

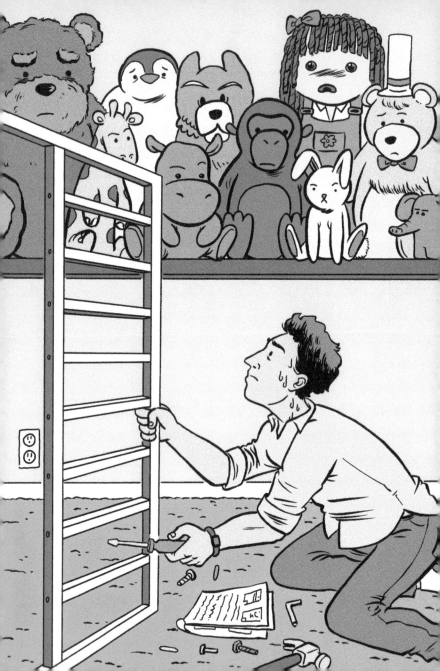

PART TWO

THE SECOND TRIMESTER

For many women, the second trimester is by far the easiest—not that *any* pregnancy stages are easy in reality. However, this period tends to find Mom getting over a lot of her early pregnancy symptoms and getting her appetite and energy back. The baby will be going through massive developmental leaps, which we will cover. One of the most exciting developments is that this trimester will reveal whether you're having a boy or a girl—that is, if you care to find out. My wife and I are planners and have always felt the need to find out so that we have as much time as possible to put together a nursery, buy clothes for the first three months, and whittle down the ol' name list. You may even entertain the idea of doing a gender reveal.

Putting a nursery together is a great opportunity for the two of you to work alongside one another and put your own creative spin on baby headquarters. And while you're out shopping for nursery furniture, bedding, and accessories, you may as well go by somewhere like Target or buybuy BABY and begin putting together a registry. We'll talk about creating a list of necessary items that will give family and friends an easy opportunity to say congratulations *and* help you stock up on everything you'll need. Also, we'll talk about when a good time would be for you and your partner to discuss a birth plan and think about touring the hospital nursery or birthing center.

There's so much happening over the next 14 weeks between doctor's appointments and fulfilling your many to-do lists. You also can't forget to talk to your individual employers about whether they offer maternity or even paternity leave. But no worries! Not only does part 2 go into more depth about all of the aforementioned, as you saw at the end of the first trimester, it includes a brief checklist that consolidates all of the important landmarks and goals to work on.

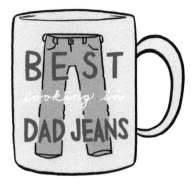

CHAPTER FOUR

The Fourth Month

Month 4 marks the beginning of the second trimester, which for many moms may be the most comfortable of all three. With any luck, a lot of the nausea and dizziness and the constant need to urinate may subside (at least temporarily). Mom's appetite and energy levels are likely to rebound, and even though her breasts have increased dramatically in size, they probably won't be as sore. Her belly will really begin looking less like she ate a huge Thanksgiving dinner and more like she's actually pregnant as the baby bump becomes more prominent.

There's a lot that we can do as future fathers throughout the entire pregnancy, but this trimester especially holds a lot of opportunities for us to do things, like establish a nursery, help Mom relax, and make a ton of lists of items both of you will need at home (or for both of your diaper bags) for when you finally bring the bambino home.

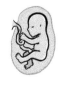

4-MONTH FETUS

NEW GEAR

neck, lanugo

SIZE COMPARISON

slightly smaller than a baseball,
dill pickle, light bulb

Making Faces

Week 14 is a big deal! Your partner has made it over the first-trimester hump (pun intended), hopefully with your love and support. Chances are that in the last week or two you made the official announcement to your friends and family, and the reactions are pouring in. It's a wonderful feeling—reconnecting with old friends and having them share their joy with you—but be wary, Pandora's box may have just been opened. Making an announcement of this magnitude (especially if you're a first-time parent) always opens up the floodgates for opinions and criticism that are not necessarily going to be welcome. Other parents (specifically moms) will most likely come forward and offer advice on every situation, so be wary of what you ask for when it comes to parenting on social media.

This week likely starts the first of the second-trimester appointments. The doctor will continue to monitor urine, blood pressure, weight, and fetal growth. Genetic testing may be an option and if she's considered high risk, insurance will generally assume the cost. Gender determination can also be included in that same test. Will it be cinnamon spice and everything nice or snips, snails, and puppy dog tails? Do you want to find out or do you prefer a surprise?

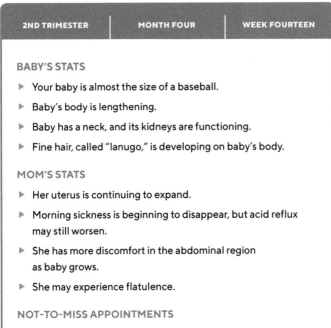

BABY'S STATS

▶ Your baby is almost the size of a baseball.

▶ Baby's body is lengthening.

▶ Baby has a neck, and its kidneys are functioning.

▶ Fine hair, called "lanugo," is developing on baby's body.

MOM'S STATS

▶ Her uterus is continuing to expand.

▶ Morning sickness is beginning to disappear, but acid reflux may still worsen.

▶ She has more discomfort in the abdominal region as baby grows.

▶ She may experience flatulence.

NOT-TO-MISS APPOINTMENTS

▶ Second-trimester appointments begin now, usually occurring every four weeks.

Hopefully, Mom is beginning to feel a little bit better and is getting over that touch of morning sickness, but she may continue to experience acid reflux. As a side note, you may want to hit the Army surplus store and grab a gas mask because her flatulence will be on the rise. Personally, it's been tough for me not to comment on occasional fart explosions from the other room over the years, and as much as I don't care and think it's funny and par for the course, it's a sensitive issue for most moms and something they wish would never happen. Maybe keep the snickers to yourself. Or if she shares your sense of humor, by all means come up with some sort of rating system so you can yell, "Hon, that was a 7.5!" from upstairs.

Family Goals

HOME CEO Begin working on the nursery: In case you haven't taken notice, Mom might be tearing apart the house, washing, drying, folding, and organizing and reorganizing the closets. This is called "nesting," and it rides shotgun with most pregnancies. At the very least, you and your partner should be talking about whether you'll have to dismantle the home office or perhaps turn the guest room into a nursery. This could take several weeks to accomplish, so don't wait until the last minute! While we're discussing this, keep in mind that Mom cannot and should not lift or push furniture or big items. Not that you're not already a gentleman, but you will need to take over the heavy lifting from here on out, so to speak.

PLAN AHEAD Inform your employer about the pregnancy: If you haven't told your employer yet, it might be wise to stop by or send an e-mail to HR, letting your company know about your partner's due date and the possibility that you might need some occasional leeway to attend checkup appointments with her physician. If your job is specialized, it would be a good idea to have some helpful suggestions about how to keep things afloat while you're out of the office. Similarly, if Mom is working outside the home, she will be having these conversations with her own employer. Maternity and paternity leave is a very pivotal experience, and you and your partner should not feel as though you can't disconnect from your professional lives and focus on your new job titles of mom and dad. Mom should check to see what kind of maternity plan her company might offer—or short-term disability might be an option in your state. In some cases, companies will offer paternity leave for dads as well. It doesn't hurt to ask; otherwise, you can save up vacation time to get some much-needed bonding time when the baby comes.

Baby Can Breathe

Mom might be able to feel the baby move this week, which is pretty magical. This is also right around the time when you'll be able to determine the gender of the baby, whether it be via ultrasound or (if your partner falls in that high-risk group of women 35 and older) genetic testing.

Along with these two momentous milestones, pay close attention whenever you see your partner set down any items of importance. For instance, car keys, cell phone, phone charger, or water bottle. I say this because one of the lesser-known side effects of having a baby is pregnancy brain. This is the condition in which your partner may misplace or lose stuff every five minutes. It's a great time to find a place in common for as many items as possible, whether it is a table when you first walk in the door, a charging station and hook, or a bowl for keys and purse. Whether or not she remembers to use such a place is the variable in this experiment! I think that I've spent as many hours searching for car keys as my wife has driven the car during each of her second trimesters.

BABY'S STATS

▶ Baby's lungs, though primitive, are functioning.

▶ Baby's legs are now longer than its arms.

▶ Your baby's taste buds have begun to develop.

MOM'S STATS

▶ Mom's belly is getting bigger.

▶ What may seem like a flutter, muscle spasm, or movement of gas in the intestines could be fetal movement.

▶ She may experience very early Braxton Hicks contractions, preparing her for childbirth.

▶ Pregnancy brain begins to kick in—resulting in brain fuzz or absentmindedness and possibly a bit of clumsiness.

▶ Psychological stress may begin to creep in—healthy baby fears. As mentioned back in Week 6, you need to stay alert for signs of prenatal mood disorders and educate yourself on the impact postpartum depression can have on new moms.

NOT-TO-MISS APPOINTMENTS

▶ If you had a second prenatal appointment and insurance didn't cover genetic testing, you may be able to schedule an ultrasound to determine the sex of the baby.

Family Goals

FUN PROJECTS Plan the gender announcement: Are you finding out and telling people the sex of the baby? I have three schools of thought on this one. First, if you and your partner consider yourself fanatical planners like my wife and I, you'll want to know as soon as possible so you can begin looking at colors of cribs, mobiles, curtains, and other nursery accessories. Knowing the sex also helps friends and family get you started with a few items before the baby comes. Second, you could wait to find out and have that awesome moment when you come into the hospital waiting room, firing off shots with your gun fingers in the air and telling everyone *it's a boy* or *it's a girl*! Or third, you and your partner could find out and keep it a secret from everyone until the delivery! We even know people who were pregnant with twins who didn't tell anyone until they met the babies. The surprise was really incredible. Due to the riches of the Internet, there are lots of ways to find inspiration for other options.

DADDY DOULA Check on weight gain: It's not a bad idea to check in with your partner about her weight gain and see if she's been advised by her doctor if she's within a healthy range.

DADDY DOULA Sign her up for a prenatal massage: A really cool and fun surprise might be to sign your partner up for one of these appointments. It shows that you care about helping her to relax and de-stress and it will probably come out of left field.

DADDY DOULA Talk about preemptively fighting the cold and flu: Mom's body is working double and triple overtime expanding her uterus and growing a baby and placenta, and this can take a toll on her immune system. Consult with your doctor about whether getting a flu shot or taking probiotics is in her best interest. And remember: Constant handwashing is a must.

PLAN AHEAD Discuss a birth plan: Does she prefer a water birth at home? Is your partner planning on having a more traditional natural birth in a hospital or birthing center? What if there are complications and an emergency C-section is required? You and your partner need to be on the *same page* (along with your doctor) in the event she's in too much pain to call the shots in the delivery room. Explore each option, decide on one, and then run through that birthing process—play devil's advocate and suggest scenarios in which you might need a plan B.

Getting Ready for a Growth Spurt

This little baby of yours is growing at an exponential rate. When I read about pregnancy status and see my wife every night after work, I feel like I'm watching Dustin take care of Dart on the second season of *Stranger Things* (though my wife is way hotter than Dart).

In other words, your baby is getting bigger by the day and is probably close to five inches long now. Its muscles are getting stronger, and Mom shouldn't be alarmed if she feels occasional movement. It can also begin responding to external stimuli, Dad. Don't be surprised if Mom can feel the baby squirm if you poke her stomach.

Family Goals

PLAN AHEAD Create a baby registry: For first-time parents, creating a baby registry can be a huge help in filling the list of things you'll need once you get the baby home from the hospital. My wife and I focused our energy on the big-ticket items in hopes that our close friends and

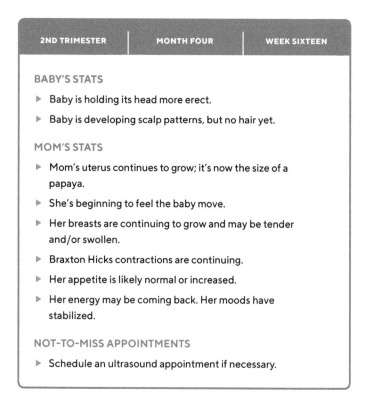

BABY'S STATS

▸ Baby is holding its head more erect.

▸ Baby is developing scalp patterns, but no hair yet.

MOM'S STATS

▸ Mom's uterus continues to grow; it's now the size of a papaya.

▸ She's beginning to feel the baby move.

▸ Her breasts are continuing to grow and may be tender and/or swollen.

▸ Braxton Hicks contractions are continuing.

▸ Her appetite is likely normal or increased.

▸ Her energy may be coming back. Her moods have stabilized.

NOT-TO-MISS APPOINTMENTS

▸ Schedule an ultrasound appointment if necessary.

extended family might be able to help us out here and there with the rest. Babies "R" Us and even Amazon are great places to start. Look at ratings on things like co-sleepers, car seats, cribs, and gliders. You certainly don't need everything that every list out there tells you to buy. And a little helpful hint: If you're planning to have more than one child, consider buying some of the larger pieces in gender-neutral colors—that way you can use them from child to child. We have pieces that my wife and I have used for all four children. During this process, hand-me-downs are also a real lifesaver, but keep in mind that certain items, such as car seats, have expiration dates (who would have thought?!).

CONVERSATION STARTERS Talk about unsolicited advice: Now that everyone knows you're pregnant, the parenting "information" or "advice" will be pouring in. You and your partner might want to talk about how to deal with that info tactfully and with grace when it's received, while (behind the scenes) picking out only what you need from that info.

CONVERSATION STARTERS Talk about belly touching: One thing that I've noticed through four pregnancies is that there's always going to be "that person" who comes on way too strong and wants to rub on that belly. So before you go off half-cocked and knock out her coworker, Jim from accounting, on a Saturday afternoon in the middle of Chipotle, you and your partner should talk about her feelings toward this sort of thing and the appropriate way to handle it. I know that my wife loved having people touch her belly—she felt it was showing love to the baby and it made her happy—but there are many women who feel the opposite. Some feel invaded no matter who is doing the touching, and it is something to really pay attention to because it's very personal to each woman.

THE ESSENTIAL BABY REGISTRY LIST

Making a baby registry can be a daunting task, especially when you have a million people in your ear telling you that "this is the absolute best" or "never buy this piece of junk, it's horrible!" My wife and I used a three-pronged strategy to figure out which product would work best for our lifestyle and situation. One, I start with online research—many mom and dad bloggers have put together somewhat unbiased lists that rate the necessities. Two, while I'm around friends who are also parents to little ones, I pay attention to some of the things they currently use and ask how they like them, along with questioning the functionality. Three, we take an afternoon or two to visit somewhere like Babies "R" Us, which does a pretty good job of making things like car seats, strollers, and cribs accessible as floor models so you can actually see how they work. I've compiled a list of essentials, in no partic-ular order: items you should consider adding to your registry in hopes that friends and family might congratulate you by helping out with necessities for life with baby.

- ☐ Infant car seat (preferably one that snaps in and out of a car adaptor and directly into a coordinated stroller)
- ☐ Stroller (with so many different models, you should get a hands-on experience if possible)
- ☐ Baby carrier (you should also test these out; moms and dads might prefer different styles, as dads might be bigger and broader)
- ☐ Layette (aka a set of newborn clothing) that covers months 0-3, 3-6, and 6-9. Aim to get the following for each three-month stage:

- ☐ 7 to 8 one-piece baby sleep-and-play outfits with footsies and built-in hand covers (get ones that zip up in the front for easy access, especially for those late-night changes)
- ☐ 5 long-sleeve onesies and 5 short-sleeve onesies (get them kimono style so you don't have to worry about messing with baby's delicate head with regular onesies)
- ☐ 5 pull-up pants (leg warmers work just as well and you don't have to take them off when changing baby)
- ☐ 2 to 3 wearable blankets
- ☐ 4 breathable muslin blankets for swaddling and other uses
- ☐ 2 hats
- ☐ 7 to 8 pairs of socks and booties
- ☐ 1 snowsuit (for the winter)

☐ Crib, mattress, mattress cover, and crib sheets (consider a three-in-one that ultimately converts into a toddler bed as baby grows)

☐ Baby monitor (a video monitor is imperative, potentially one that connects to your smartphone)

☐ Bottles, a breast pump if breastfeeding, and formula if not breastfeeding

☐ Bibs and burp cloths

☐ Newborn-size disposable or cloth diapers and wipes

☐ Diaper Genie (or some sort of system to contain those *many* diapers you're about to change)

☐ Baby bathtub and toiletries

☐ Baby first aid kit, rectal thermometer, and nail clippers

☐ Baby bouncer

A Little Baby Fat

Your baby is accumulating a ton of subcutaneous fat this week as it continues to grow at a rapid rate. The baby is the size of a pomegranate, *and* one of the coolest things that more than likely goes down this week is they can begin to hear you.

So grab your tap shoes, top hat, cane, and whatever old theater props you have left over from high school or college and warm up the living room stage to offer some entertainment for this little developing mind. Or if you're like me, after your partner goes to sleep, you'll be putting Bose headphones over her stomach and shuffling stand-up routines from some of your favorite comics through iTunes.

Family Goals

DADDY DOULA Sign up for childbirth classes: My wife and I never got around to taking these, but I wish that we would have. These classes will prepare you and your partner for labor and birth with a series of lessons, discussions, and exercises.

BABY'S STATS

- ▶ Baby's bones are getting stronger as they harden from cartilage.
- ▶ Baby is beginning to develop sweat glands.
- ▶ The umbilical cord is strengthening and thickening.

MOM'S STATS

- ▶ Mom's belly continues to grow, and her center of gravity is shifting, which may make her clumsier.
- ▶ Pregnancy brain is in full effect.
- ▶ Her blood flow is increasing, as are flows of other fluids in her body. She may have the occasional bloody nose. She's also gaining weight more rapidly than before.
- ▶ As her skin stretches, she may notice itching all over her body. Lotion or coconut oil may be a helpful remedy. (I buy my wife coconut oil because it doesn't have a fragrance and is natural.)

NOT-TO-MISS APPOINTMENTS

- ▶ If the first second-trimester appointment hasn't happened yet, then make an appointment this week.

PREGNANCY EMPATHY 101 Be patient with momnesia: Small bouts of forgetfulness are common when she tries to find her keys, phone, purse, shoes, and so forth.

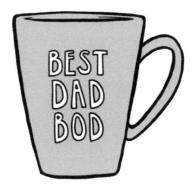

CHAPTER FIVE

The Fifth Month

Mom's belly is getting rounder and rounder, and even though you're already entering the fifth month, for some reason, it may just be beginning to hit home that this is the real deal. She'll begin to feel little flutters and movement inside of her tummy, which is an emotionally comforting feeling— she's finally getting a constant reminder that there's a baby on the way.

Aside from doctor's appointments every month to check on Mom's and baby's health, you'll also get to visit with the little one via an ultrasound. Between the ultrasound and any genetic testing, you'll have the option to find out if it's a boy or a girl!

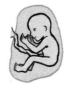

5-MONTH FETUS

NEW GEAR

genitals, ears, vernix on skin

SIZE COMPARISON

Belgian endive, paper airplane, Choco Taco

Gender!

Up until the 1970s, when ultrasound equipment advanced and got sharp enough to identify genitals, there really was no way to find out ahead of time whether you and your partner were having a boy or a girl. There were no fancy gender reveals—you simply trudged out to the waiting room in your operating room scrubs and booties and hoped that a handful of folks were still there to hug you, stick a cigar in your pocket, possibly take a picture, visit Mom in recovery, and see the baby through the glass of the nursery. With the advent of improved technology and social media, many couples will either find out in the doctor's office *or* have the OB/GYN write it down in a sealed envelope to be revealed in some other way.

My wife and I started off slowly: With our first baby, we found out in the doctor's office, and shared the news with our parents. With our second, we got more creative and had our doctor write down the sex in a sealed envelope, which we handed over to a baker, who had instructions to make the cake with completely hidden pink or blue insides and thick white fondant icing. We invited our family and friends over and found out alongside them that we were having a boy. With our third, we had the doctor write down the gender, and my wife and I shared a private meal

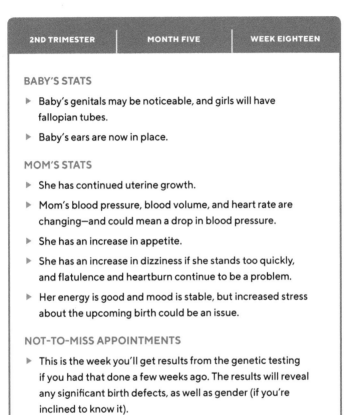

BABY'S STATS

- ► Baby's genitals may be noticeable, and girls will have fallopian tubes.
- ► Baby's ears are now in place.

MOM'S STATS

- ► She has continued uterine growth.
- ► Mom's blood pressure, blood volume, and heart rate are changing—and could mean a drop in blood pressure.
- ► She has an increase in appetite.
- ► She has an increase in dizziness if she stands too quickly, and flatulence and heartburn continue to be a problem.
- ► Her energy is good and mood is stable, but increased stress about the upcoming birth could be an issue.

NOT-TO-MISS APPOINTMENTS

- ► This is the week you'll get results from the genetic testing if you had that done a few weeks ago. The results will reveal any significant birth defects, as well as gender (if you're inclined to know it).

together and discovered the sex privately. We then planned a reveal for the kids, family, and Internet crowd—stuffing colored balloons into a box and opening it in a field. Most recently with pregnancy number four, we found the company Poof There It Is!

that designs CO_2-powered chalk cannons that you can twist, and footballs and golf balls that you can throw or hit, that reveal the gender in a massive brightly colored cloud of powder. Any way you cut it, Pinterest or Instagram will surely have the next trendy way to make your announcement.

Family Goals

CONVERSATION STARTERS Decide on the gender reveal: If you're receiving genetic testing results or your ultrasound revealed the answer, this is the perfect time to finish that conversation (before you get on the phone to hear the results) about whether you and your partner want to be informed about the gender and if you're planning on sharing it and how.

DAD RD Stock up on her favorite snacks: With Mom's appetite lit, keep that pantry stacked with her favorite (somewhat healthy) snacks.

STRESS REDUCER Take her to the movies: The stress continues to mount. Take your partner out to a movie to take her mind off of things.

Sensory Development

Your baby's senses are in full development now within the brain, which may also coincide with a growth spurt, so keep your eyes peeled for Mom swiping food off of your plate when you get up to use the restroom. A little bigger than a mango, your baby is also covered in something called *vernix caseosa*, a substance similar to the Nickelodeon Kids' Choice Awards slime, except this slime is white. It's a greasy substance that covers your baby's sensitive skin, protecting it from that long soak in the amniotic bath. Don't worry, unless premature, most babies lose this coating at birth—no need to break out the pressure washer.

As the chance of leg cramps or hip pain increases, don't be afraid if your partner lets out a shriek in the middle of the night—she's overcome by the infamous charley horse. If you happen to wake up (and can talk through your sleep apnea mask), advise her to point her toes upward, and the stress should begin to relieve.

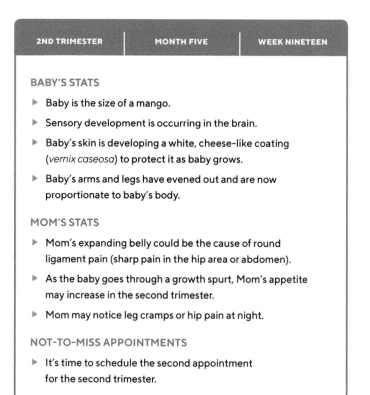

BABY'S STATS

▶ Baby is the size of a mango.

▶ Sensory development is occurring in the brain.

▶ Baby's skin is developing a white, cheese-like coating (*vernix caseosa*) to protect it as baby grows.

▶ Baby's arms and legs have evened out and are now proportionate to baby's body.

MOM'S STATS

▶ Mom's expanding belly could be the cause of round ligament pain (sharp pain in the hip area or abdomen).

▶ As the baby goes through a growth spurt, Mom's appetite may increase in the second trimester.

▶ Mom may notice leg cramps or hip pain at night.

NOT-TO-MISS APPOINTMENTS

▶ It's time to schedule the second appointment for the second trimester.

Family Goals

DADDY DOULA Buy her a maternity pillow: Mom's uterus is continuing to expand and the baby is growing like mad, which means it might be difficult for her to find a comfortable sleeping position. If she's hasn't already purchased one (or you didn't pull the old one down from the attic), consider a sleep aid for Mom (no, not chloroform) or perhaps a wedge or long pillow. Personally, I've given up a decent percentage of our king bed to something called the "Snoogle." Go ahead, look it up. It may take some in-store testing to determine if a circular or triangular wedge pillow *or* a flexible U-shaped or L-shaped configuration is best.

BROWNIE POINTS Get your honorary masseuse license: Mom's legs and hips may be beginning to hurt; offer to lightly massage them to relieve any cramping.

Halfway There

You're at the midpoint of 40 weeks, basically halfway to the birth of your child. The baby is roughly the length of a banana and the width of a small artichoke. This is a big week for gender development. If it's a girl, her uterus is formed and her ovaries are holding about 7 million primitive eggs (though this will drop significantly by birth), and her vaginal canal is formed. If it's a boy, his testicles have hopped in the car and are heading down south toward the abdomen for spring break! Give it a few more months, and they'll officially stop sleeping in the car and move into the scrotum (that's still under construction). The UFC title match in Mom's belly that includes twisting, turning, cartwheels, and roundhouse kicks is just starting to heat up—you may want to pull up a seat next to your partner and get ready to do some consoling.

Family Goals

BONDING TIME Celebrate: A lot of couples don't actually realize that they've hit the midpoint of pregnancy because they're so focused on trimesters. This is a

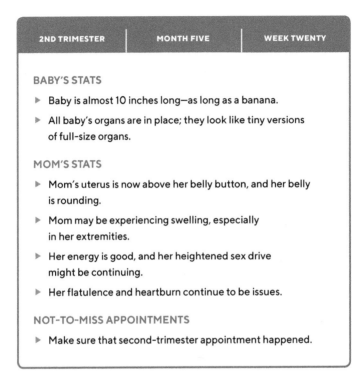

BABY'S STATS

- Baby is almost 10 inches long—as long as a banana.
- All baby's organs are in place; they look like tiny versions of full-size organs.

MOM'S STATS

- Mom's uterus is now above her belly button, and her belly is rounding.
- Mom may be experiencing swelling, especially in her extremities.
- Her energy is good, and her heightened sex drive might be continuing.
- Her flatulence and heartburn continue to be issues.

NOT-TO-MISS APPOINTMENTS

- Make sure that second-trimester appointment happened.

great opportunity or excuse to go and grab dinner together. Celebrate! You're halfway (or less) to the finish line.

FUN PROJECTS Choose potential baby names: While you're out to dinner celebrating the halfway point, share your top three boy or girl names with each other, and why they're important to you.

Kung Fu Fighting

Your baby is closing in on a foot in length and a pound in weight. The good news is that hopefully Mom is not feeling as bad as she was during that first trimester, and her appetite should be almost completely back to normal. One thing to note is that the flavor of amniotic fluid varies from day to day depending on what she's eaten. So in theory, you've got a decent chance of your baby liking things like carrots and whatever is on your menu because they are swallowing this amniotic fluid not only for hydration but for nutrition as well. Another thing to keep in mind is that the baby's arms and legs are now finally in proportion, so the punches and kicks will be much more coordinated movements, rather than the herky-jerky moves Mom has felt up until now.

BABY'S STATS

▶ Your baby is as long as a carrot and as thick as an endive.

▶ Baby's eyebrows have grown in.

▶ Females are developing a vagina.

MOM'S STATS

▶ Mom's body has increased oil production, and progesterone level is increasing.

▶ Pressure on the bladder and legs is also increasing.

▶ Complaints such as nausea, dizziness, and overall fatigue have decreased or disappeared altogether.

▶ Her mood is upbeat and energy is high.

▶ She could get varicose or spider veins.

NOT-TO-MISS APPOINTMENTS

▶ Ask the doctor about preeclampsia, as this is a typical week when symptoms might appear.

Family Goals

DADDY DOULA Help Mom steer clear of varicose veins: These veins are common in the lower half of the body during pregnancy as women produce an extra volume of blood. Encourage her to keep her legs uncrossed while watching TV at night, keep moving during the day, and maybe even sleep on her left side when possible—this avoids putting pressure on the main blood vessels and keeps circulation moving.

BROWNIE POINTS Go shoe shopping: Not for yourself, but for Mom. She has more than likely given up the highest of her high heels, and her new best friend is about to become flats. It could be a great idea to find out what brand she likes (like Tieks or Toms) and surprise her with a pair! (Note: You may want to do some investigating, as some women will go up a half size during pregnancy. Also, consider flats without laces because bending over to tie shoes is a feat all its own.)

A Very Tiny Baby

Your baby is now a full one-pounder and a feisty one at that.
Baby is more than likely touching and grabbing the umbilical
cord and is able to notice things like loud music, sirens, and dogs
barking, and may even be light sensitive—if you put a flashlight
up to Mommy's belly, he or she may turn away as a response.
This little softball is only a week or two away from being viable
if born premature. Hopefully, you were able to find some sort
of sleep aid in the form of a pillow; Mom is going to need it.

Family Goals

DADDY DOULA Check Mom's vitals: Ask your partner
how she's feeling. Many women will have hot flashes
or constantly feel like they're sweating. Cool showers, cold
compresses, or even snacking on frozen fruit may help bring
the body temperature down. My wife often feels dizzy during
her pregnancies, and often this is due to dehydration or possibly low blood sugar. Remind your partner to keep up her
water intake, as well as to keep snacking throughout the day
so she doesn't pass out!

BABY'S STATS

▶ Baby is the size of a papaya and a week or two away from being viable should Mom go into premature labor.

▶ Baby truly looks like a little skinny baby.

▶ Baby's pancreas has developed.

▶ Baby's irises are there, but are colorless.

▶ Baby will break the one-pound barrier this week!

MOM'S STATS

▶ Mom is noticing baby moving throughout the day.

▶ Mom's belly is clearly a pregnant one at this point.

▶ She may have pigment changes in her skin or a dark line running up the middle of her belly.

▶ She'll experience an increase in discomfort as baby continues to grow.

▶ She may have difficulty finding a comfortable position for sleeping.

▶ Her poor sleep, heartburn, and flatulence may cause stress.

NOT-TO-MISS APPOINTMENTS

▶ Follow up on the third second-trimester appointment.

CONVERSATION STARTERS Discuss breastfeeding with Mom and what you can do to help: Is this something that she plans on doing once the baby is born? If it's something Mom wants to do, encourage her to research nursing bras and styled shirts that are easy to nurse with: She might want to start wearing these a couple of weeks before going to the hospital to break them in a bit. In addition, you might look into a portable breast pump that she'll be able to take with her while at work or on the road. Check with your insurance, as a breast pump could be available free of charge!

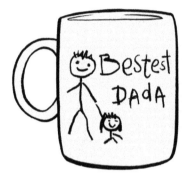

CHAPTER SIX

The Sixth Month

This month marks the end of the second trimester, which means that you're two-thirds of the way to meeting your baby for the first time. As the baby continues to grow and get stronger, those arms and legs will be flapping and kicking away, which means that they will make more of an impact on the inside of the uterus, packing a heavier punch. The baby is furiously gaining weight and beginning to add fat to its loose skin.

Mom should be resting whenever she can, continuing to eat healthy, and getting plenty of water and fluids. The baby is eating and drinking everything that Mom is, and Mom needs to keep that in mind as she moves through her daily routine.

You should be kicking into high gear this month, continuing to help with household responsibilities as much as possible—as Mom continues to get bigger and bigger, it will become harder for her to do some of the simple things she was accustomed to.

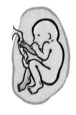

6-MONTH FETUS

NEW GEAR

fat development

SIZE COMPARISON

G.I. Joe action figure, Pringles can

NOTES

opens eyes, sucks thumb, hiccups,
recognizes sounds and voices

Packing on the Pounds

The second trimester to me always felt like the garbage time at the end of a football game, with teams going through the motions to run out the clock and the winning team celebrating the inevitable. Most of the baby's essential parts are fully developed and moving forward; it's a big job to keep packing on the pounds. Your baby is about the size of a grapefruit wearing a suit of saggy skin that will soon be filled out. Skin grows quicker than the baby can stuff it with fat, but that will change over the next few weeks.

Mom's mood is probably pretty good, although the two of you have a lot of planning (and executing) to do before the delivery date. Now is the perfect time to think about items that you'll need for a diaper bag. My wife ditched her small purse and went to a bigger, trendy designer bag that doubled as both her purse *and* diaper bag.

BABY'S STATS

▶ Blood vessels in baby's lungs are developing as it prepares to breathe outside the womb.

▶ Baby is adding fat.

MOM'S STATS

▶ Baby is pushing Mom's liver upward and her belly is growing outward.

▶ Mom may notice a bit of water retention and swelling in her feet and/or legs.

▶ Mom's mood is even and upbeat even though she is struggling with the physical discomforts associated with this stage of pregnancy.

▶ Her appetite is hearty.

▶ Eating smaller amounts at each sitting can help alleviate the continuing flatulence, bloating, and heartburn.

NOT-TO-MISS APPOINTMENTS

▶ Absent special concerns, the third second-trimester appointment will be more of the same.

Family Goals

☑ PLAN AHEAD Shopping for baby essentials: Although Mom has probably already begun collecting items necessary for the nursery, now is a perfect time to double-check your birth registry list and check off the remaining boxes. Divvy up the list by concentrating on the stuff you are most interested in. If you're anything like me, you'll want to volunteer to research the techy stuff, such as the baby monitor/camera, music, white-noise machine, and night-light, and now is a great time to do it. Mom may prefer to focus more on the crib (will you get a three-in-one transitional crib?), the bedding, and the comfort factor of a glider or rocking nursing chair. Note: You may want to make your second, follow-up trip to finalize exactly what you like.

☑ PLAN AHEAD Buy a diaper bag: While Mom is picking out her own diaper bag, you may want to consider getting your own messenger-style diaper bag. Or if you're anything like me, look for a backpack designed especially for dads (there are a bunch out there now) with a military or more rugged feel to them—such as Madpax, Jack Spade, or Diaper Dude. During our first pregnancy, my guy friends surprised me with a dad's diaper bag (a camo messenger bag). But then I switched over to a backpack for our second child and never looked back. It's all about personal preference and ultimately the functionality that works for you.

Viability!

Breathe easy: This is a huge week mentally for you and Mom.
You've achieved that viability marker. Half to three-fourths of
all babies born this week survive, and with each passing day, the
survival rate increases. This is significant because it helps lessen
the load of stress on you and, most importantly, on Mom. If
your baby was born this week, it would have a face that looked
like a face, with eyelashes, eyebrows, hair, and every other fully
developed part.

The baby is still accumulating baby fat and strengthening
those organs, bones, and muscle. If you're wondering whether
your baby will be a blonde, brunette, or redhead, you can keep
guessing—the hair pigment isn't there yet.

Mom is continuing to experience all the good stuff: lower back
pain, trouble sleeping, heartburn, whoopee cushion-caliber flatulence (beware of the Dutch oven at night), and the unfortunate
swelling of the limbs. Encourage your partner to kick her feet
up and rest whenever possible, stay hydrated, and continue her
healthy eating habits.

BABY'S STATS

▶ Baby is the length of an ear of corn, about one foot long.

▶ Baby's lungs are formed, and baby is now strong enough that it has a 50 to 75 percent chance of surviving outside the womb.

MOM'S STATS

▶ Mom's uterus is now the size of a soccer ball.

▶ She may have back pain, difficulty sleeping, heartburn, flatulence, and swelling.

NOT-TO-MISS APPOINTMENTS

▶ Check with your doctor about when a test for gestational diabetes (aka pregnancy diabetes) should be scheduled. This is also referred to as a "glucose test" and the results can usually be determined during the scheduled visit. (My wife tells me the test is kind of like drinking an extra-strong batch of Crush soda but having your blood checked before and after.)

GESTATIONAL DIABETES

One of the tests or screenings that Mom may have to endure (if basic urine screenings reveal high sugar content) is the glucose test for gestational diabetes. She drinks a thick, sugary liquid and is given a blood test. If the test reveals that she has gestational diabetes, she'll have to work with her doctor to determine how out of whack her glucose levels might be and find a diet that helps maintain a balance. Dad can help by keeping Mom on track with what she's eating and taking that into consideration while preparing meals.

Family Goals

PLAN AHEAD Pack your hospital bags: These bags will be lifesavers and are 100 percent necessary to have packed in the event that the baby comes before you were expecting it!

DADDY DOULA Learn the signs of pre-labor: The baby suddenly drops, your partner has her water break, she experiences severe signs of lower back pain or contractions, and she has diarrhea/nausea or bloody vaginal discharge. If you see these signs, it's time to put on your game face, call your doctor, and grab that bag that you (hopefully) packed for the hospital.

HOSPITAL BAG CHECKLIST

I've experienced a few different hospitals, and the setup is generally the same. Once Mom is moved to recovery, there will be a pull-out sofa or a cot for Dad to sleep in. It's generally no-frills, and you may want to consider packing comfort items in your bags. Many of these rooms have their own shower, and it'll feel good after a long night to rinse off before heading down to the cafeteria to grab a meal. Here are a few essentials (the contents of her bags and mine were similar).

- ☐ A few days' worth of extra-comfortable clothes (sweatpants, hoodies—Mom needs to bring tops that keep her breasts easily accessible for nursing and also, in case of a C-section, loose-fitting pants that don't fit low across her incision)
- ☐ Water bottles
- ☐ GoPro or video recording equipment and chargers
- ☐ Laptop or tablet with downloaded movies or a TV series
- ☐ Kindle or book
- ☐ Phone chargers
- ☐ Dopp kit (hygiene items you would take on any overnight trip)
- ☐ Sleeping pad (for Dad—a blow-up camping pad may feel better than the worn cot mattress springs)
- ☐ Feminine pads (for Mom—the hospital will generally supply Mom with more than enough, but it can never hurt to have extra)
- ☐ "Mom underwear" (Sorry guys, don't expect to be seeing her in a thong too soon, and say hello to full-coverage undies: It's a necessity both for comfort and to hold the feminine pads that are larger than your newborn's diapers.)

Losing Wrinkles

Your baby weighs around 1½ **pounds** and measures almost 13 inches long—not quite Shaq's basketball sneaker but getting there. It's roughly the size of an acorn squash, or if you're sick of taking a tour through produce, a small chuck roast.

The baby continues to gain weight and is filling its body with fat. Capillaries are forming under the skin and filling with blood—at the end of this week, air sacs lined with capillaries will also develop in your baby's lungs, getting them ready for their first breath of air. Keep in mind, they won't be able to completely function on their own—they still need a bit more maturing. Mom is trudging along, and the same things that have taxed her over the last few weeks continue to persist.

Family Goals

DAD RD Experiment with tapas: At this point in the pregnancy, it might be difficult for Mom to eat big meals. If you're making dinner, consider making a small sampling of a few different items—maybe even including sautéed spinach to give her that important iron that she might need.

BABY'S STATS

▶ Baby is adding fat and filling out.

▶ Baby's hair begins to pigment.

▶ Baby's skin is dewrinkling.

MOM'S STATS

▶ Mom's growing uterus is putting pressure on the vessels leading to her lower extremities, which is causing swelling, particularly in warm weather.

▶ Discomfort and trouble sleeping can continue to be an issue.

▶ This is a great week to add iron to her diet if she's anemic— check with the doctor.

▶ Small meals can alleviate heartburn.

NOT-TO-MISS APPOINTMENTS

▶ If the third second-trimester appointment has occurred, check on the test for iron-deficiency anemia, particularly if she's feeling run down or tired.

▶ If you haven't already discussed a birth center, hospital, or birth plan with your doctor, this is a great time.

PLAN AHEAD Revisit and finalize a birth plan: Assuming that you and your partner have already determined your birth plan, this would be a great time to revisit and refresh, including whether an epidural might be necessary and at what time. Also, begin researching an official doula, a birth companion aside from you, who helps provide physical, mental, and emotional support throughout the pregnancy and postpartum. Her role isn't to replace you as a husband or partner but rather to work in tandem with you to make this time as easy as possible for your partner. Also, make sure to look at your budget and see if this is financially feasible.

The Descending Testicles

If you're having a boy, this is the week that testicles are descending into the now fully formed scrotum. Your baby is almost two pounds now, the size of an average chuck roast, and is close to 14 inches long. After several weeks of having its eyelids fused together to allow the retina to develop, your baby's eyes are beginning to open. The iris (the colored part of the eye) doesn't have pigmentation yet, but it will soon.

My wife begins experiencing heartburn *really* early in her pregnancies, and if heartburn hasn't reared its head already, it can probably be expected any day. It gives her a strong esophageal burning feeling along with the sensation that she can't catch her breath. This symptom, along with the growing discomfort of her expanding stomach, can contribute to a lack of sleep and an irritable disposition.

BABY'S STATS

- ▶ Baby's senses are developing.
- ▶ Baby's lungs are continuing to strengthen.
- ▶ Baby weighs around two pounds and can open its eyes.
- ▶ If it's a boy, the testicles are descending.

MOM'S STATS

- ▶ As Mom's belly continues to swell, her center of gravity has shifted and is causing issues with sleeping and overall discomfort.
- ▶ Her physical discomfort and a lack of sleep can be making Mom irritable.
- ▶ Braxton Hicks contractions are continuing as she prepares for birth.
- ▶ Her heartburn is worsening.
- ▶ Her clumsiness continues, especially when getting up after being seated for a long time.

NOT-TO-MISS APPOINTMENTS

- ▶ The second-trimester appointments continue as scheduled.

Family Goals

STRESS REDUCER Schedule a third-trimester pregnancy massage: To alleviate some of that stress and physical discomfort that's sure to increase as your partner prepares for the homestretch, scheduling a pregnancy massage (with enough notice to cancel without penalty) for your partner might be a swell idea to put her mind (and body) at ease.

PREGNANCY EMPATHY 101 Read up on Braxton Hicks contractions: These are known as prodromal labor or "practice contractions." These contractions are essentially a feeling of false labor that can start as early as Week 6 and continue well into the second and third trimesters. Talk to your partner about how she feels, and see if there's any way you can make her feel more comfortable when they arise.

The End of the Second Trimester

Getting through the second trimester is an exciting time: You're two-thirds of the way into this journey together. Considering all the baby stats, this hasn't been the easiest trimester for Mom. Your baby is definitely displaying distinct baby qualities, including its insane sense of taste. It can differentiate between the taste of amniotic fluid and other things that Mom is eating. In fact, your baby has more taste buds now than it will have at birth and beyond. Many moms notice distinct reactions from baby when eating specific foods.

My wife has a penchant for spicy foods, and there's little or no chance that I'm standing in between her and that jar of sliced jalapeños in our refrigerator. However, that doesn't mean that I won't remind her of the aftereffects. In her first three pregnancies, she experienced several restless nights of the baby kicking and experiencing the hiccups, trying to shake the aftertaste of her 10,000-Scoville dinner.

There might be a few other things that pop up (or out) around this time, including her belly button. If your partner had a piercing, it's no problem to keep it in—unless it begins to poke

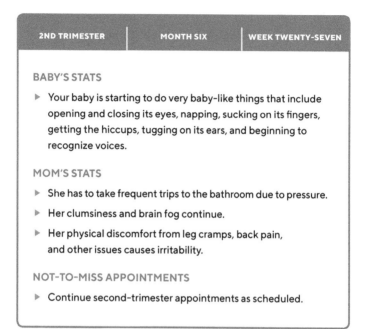

BABY'S STATS

▶ Your baby is starting to do very baby-like things that include opening and closing its eyes, napping, sucking on its fingers, getting the hiccups, tugging on its ears, and beginning to recognize voices.

MOM'S STATS

▶ She has to take frequent trips to the bathroom due to pressure.

▶ Her clumsiness and brain fog continue.

▶ Her physical discomfort from leg cramps, back pain, and other issues causes irritability.

NOT-TO-MISS APPOINTMENTS

▶ Continue second-trimester appointments as scheduled.

through the shirts she's wearing or tends to get caught on her wardrobe. If that is the case, simply take the jewelry out and reinsert it every few days to make sure the hole doesn't close. Look into belly button covers that are used to keep that bad boy at bay.

And if the stretching has gotten to the point where she's complaining about a constantly itchy tummy, ditch the lotion and go for something thicker such as coconut oil—this is what my wife uses (I also give it a spin on my own stomach after Thanksgiving dinner)—or any kind of shea or belly butter. Any of these should calm the itch down right away!

Family Goals

CONVERSATION STARTERS Book a doula (or not): If that's the road you're thinking about, it's probably time for an interview and meet and greet. You may also want to ask other moms or parents in your area what type of compensation a doula might be looking for.

DAD RD Monitor rest and nutrition goals: Has your partner been keeping a journal of her sleep activity and meals? It's never too late to begin keeping track of this stuff; in fact, there are apps that can do some of the heavy lifting for you. Sprout is a great option for moms and the fatherhood community *The Life of Dad* has rolled out an "Expecting" page and app for their website, written by men, for men.

THE SECOND-TRIMESTER CHECKLIST

HOME:

☐ Begin working on the nursery.

☐ Create a baby registry with your partner (see page 98 for The Essential Baby Registry List).

BABY:

☐ Sign up for childbirth and Lamaze classes.

☐ Plan the gender reveal with your partner.

☐ Share some baby names that you like with your partner.

MOM:

☐ Buy a maternity pillow and flat shoes to help your partner be comfortable and feel cared for.

☐ At this point in the pregnancy it will be tough for Mom to eat large meals. Focus on cooking her smaller samplings of a few different items.

☐ Discuss breastfeeding with your partner and the baby's doctor.

PRENATAL APPOINTMENTS:

☐ Between 18 and 20 weeks, fetal ultrasound will reveal gender and allow the doctor to examine baby's major developments.

☐ Around 24 weeks, glucose screening test

HOSPITAL:

☐ Discuss the birth plan with your partner.

☐ Start packing your hospital bags. It's never too early to be ready.

☐ Talk with your partner about whether you want to hire a doula or not. If you do, begin gathering referrals and interviewing potential candidates.

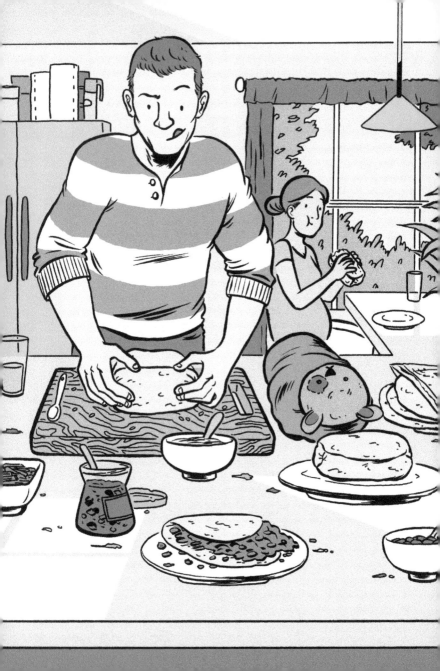

PART THREE

THE THIRD TRIMESTER

Dude. You're in the final stretch! You're two-thirds of the way there and almost to the finish line.

The third trimester starts off on a *very* positive note. Baby's viability increases to close to 100 percent if born prematurely. This takes a lot of stress off both parents, but especially Mom.

Mom is feeling more and more discomfort as the days go by. The baby is growing at an exponential rate inside the uterus, stretching Mom and her tummy to the limit. Everything will eventually become difficult for her as we creep toward the delivery date.

Baby is filling out its saggy skin and gaining the fat it will need to live outside the womb. It will also be punching, kicking, turning, and churning like it's in an all-out street brawl in Mom's belly.

This trimester is a key opportunity for Dad to step up and tie the bow on all of those loose-end projects that need to be completed before the baby comes home. Putting together a crib, moving furniture, painting the nursery (Mom can't be around the fumes), and hopefully continuing to escort Mom to her doctor's appointments can really show her how much you care about being a partner and a player during this pregnancy, instead of just watching from the bench.

We'll talk about interviewing pediatricians and finalizing a birth plan together with your partner. And if you ever thought about taking childbirth classes, this is also a great thing to do as a couple. Don't forget, finding *and* installing a car seat is something you won't want to wait until the last minute to do, and there's a certain art behind putting together a his-and-hers hospital bag. Buckle up for the final few laps, because you're about to become a father!

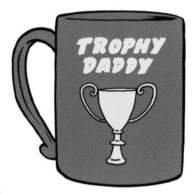

CHAPTER SEVEN

The Seventh Month

Six months down and only three to go! This is the beginning of the third trimester, and things are about to get hot and *heavy*. When I say heavy, I mean that this trimester is all about the baby finishing up development of bones and organs and adding much-needed fat to survive. This growth only begins to crowd Mom's uterus, and those basic daily tasks begin to become much more difficult.

This month is important for many reasons, but mainly because if your baby was born prematurely, it would have a 96 percent survival rate, which is a wonderful piece of information.

Your baby is developing its brain and is finally able to turn its head.

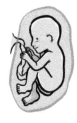

7-MONTH FETUS

NEW GEAR

forehead, bone marrow/development of red cells

SIZE COMPARISON

pineapple, a roller skate, bottle of whisky

NOTES

smiles, kicks, punches, moves head side to side,
flips, experiences REM sleep, and dreams

A Jump in Viability

Babies born at 28 weeks have an incredible 96 percent survival rate. It's still ideal that they reach full term, but this is just a great statistic to have at this point. The baby is more than likely moving into a head-down position to get ready for birth. Despite this good news, Mom is having a lot of discomfort these days, with the size and weight of the baby causing back pain and pressing on the sciatic nerve.

I always playfully referred to my wife as "the director" as she went into the third trimester. I didn't want her lifting any heavy items or climbing up on 10-foot ladders to change lightbulbs. I always insisted that she relax and make herself comfortable, and I'd take over on the projects that still needed attention.

If your baby area or nursery isn't complete, now is a great time for the both of you to pick out paint samples, order or hang a mobile, assemble the crib, and look into possibly getting a nursing chair for the corner—something that is able to rock or sway back and forth. This helps not only with nursing but also if it's Dad's turn to feed the baby or rock the baby back to sleep at 3 a.m. so Mom can catch up on some much-needed rest.

For my wife and me, this was an important purchase, one that we wanted to buy gender neutral so we could use it for all of our

BABY'S STATS

▶ Baby weighs about 2¼ pounds and is the size of a small eggplant.

▶ Baby's lungs are maturing.

▶ Baby is hopefully moving into the head-down position, preparing to be born in a few short months.

▶ Baby's brain is developing rapidly by growing neurons.

▶ This is a huge week, as baby's chance of surviving outside the womb if born premature is now 96 percent.

MOM'S STATS

▶ Her internal organs are becoming squished.

▶ Baby's increased movements mean that Mom is feeling kicks and wiggles more frequently.

▶ She's likely experiencing frequent backaches and sciatic pain as the baby begins to press on the sciatic nerve.

▶ She may have shortness of breath as baby presses up into her lungs.

NOT-TO-MISS APPOINTMENTS

▶ Third-trimester appointments now shift to every two weeks instead of every four. If your doctor hasn't mentioned it before, they may recommend STD testing, as some STDs can cause complications at birth. If Rh testing was negative, the doctor will begin immunoglobulin injections.

babies. Eight years later we are glad we splurged and bought the Little Castle glider. It has held up really well and will even be able to be passed down to our grandchildren someday.

Family Goals

DADDY DOULA Help Mom relieve sciatica: There are several stretches that can help relieve pressure on the sciatic nerve. The table stretch and pigeon pose are two great ways to ease the pain.

PLAN AHEAD Take another look at your lists: Have you filled all the basic needs for your nursery? For your diaper bags? Your hospital bag? Have you gone to Babies "R" Us or buybuy BABY and tested out car seats that will snap into all of your cars as well as a stroller to make your lives so much easier while running errands or traveling? The fancy-schmancy jogging strollers are great—we've had about five different brands from Bumbleride to Quinny—but in the first couple of months you need a Snap 'n Go or a similar stroller so you don't have to remove the baby from his or her seat every time you get in and out of the vehicle. These strollers are literally just frames that the car seat snaps into. One of these makes your life much easier, and besides, who wants to wake a sleeping baby?

Smiling on the Inside

The baby is continuing to grow and gain weight and at this point is probably 15 to 16 inches long and around 2½ to 3 pounds. It is beginning to experience REM sleep during its sleeping cycles. Because the baby is growing so quickly, it's beginning to get cramped in there, and instead of forceful kicks or punches, Mom will probably begin to feel softer blows that are more like jabs and pokes instead. The other wonderful surprise that might happen around this time is a dampening of the breasts. Mom's body is producing prolactin, which can cause the release of colostrum from the nipples.

Family Goals

PLAN AHEAD Interview a pediatrician: Crowdsource or ask friends with kids for referrals to local pediatricians. You can do a lot of research online, but most pediatricians will take a few minutes to sit down with you and your partner and discuss their practice to see if it aligns with your beliefs.

BABY'S STATS

▶ Baby has started smiling and is the size of a butternut squash.

▶ Baby is entering episodes of REM sleep and possibly dreaming.

▶ Baby's bones are mineralizing (hardening).

▶ The forehead is bulging with a growing brain.

▶ Baby's current weight is going to double, triple, and more over the next three months.

MOM'S STATS

▶ Mom's body is producing more prolactin in anticipation of lactation.

▶ Her belly is growing larger and rounder.

▶ Her fundal height may be as much as four inches above the naval.

▶ Her urination has gone from frequent to all the time.

▶ Her grace in movement has gone out the window.

▶ Colostrum may begin to release from her breasts.

NOT-TO-MISS APPOINTMENTS

▶ Mom is having doctor's appointments every two weeks now that we're in the third trimester, so she should have one this week. See Week 28 for details.

DADDY DOULA Help Mom find the bathroom: With the uterus getting filled up, the baby is constantly pressing on Mom's bladder, so she'll be urinating early, often, and always. I'm always helping my wife scout for the nearest bathroom when we jump from errand to errand on a Saturday or try a restaurant for the first time. This isn't the best time to get stuck in a long line somewhere or underestimate the duration of a gentle weekend nature walk—unless Mom is comfortable dropping trou in public.

DADDY DOULA Carry backup clothing: It's always a solid idea to have a backup shirt, sweater, or jacket within reach. It might even be a good idea for your partner to look into having breast pads handy to avoid a potentially awkward shopping situation. There's nothing like walking around Target with two wet spots in conspicuous locations!

BONDING TIME Enroll in childbirth classes: I've mentioned this once before, and it's not too late to look into taking a few classes before the big day. Again, this is something you can do *together* and something that will bring you closer in the process. Lamaze, childcare 101, and baby CPR are great alternative classes as well.

Your Little Cabbage

Your baby is about 16 inches long and close to three pounds at this point. Its brain is rapidly forming, including all of those grooves and creases that will provide much-needed room to expand as baby makes the jump from helpless newborn to responsive infant to verbal toddler to out-of-control pre-schooler (I've got one of those) and beyond (two of those!).

Your baby's brain is taking on different tasks now as well. For the past several weeks, your baby has been covered in fine, silk-like hairs (lanugo) that helped keep it warm. But now the baby's brain is able to do that, so that lanugo is slowly disappearing, and at birth it will most likely be gone.

Mom's ligaments are relaxing in preparation for the baby's birth, and the size of the baby and uterus are causing all kinds of discomfort. Her feet are widening too, but take it from me, don't be too quick to call her "sasquatch foot" unless you want to get kicked into next week. Instead, rub those beasts while you're sitting together on the sofa watching a newly released romcom.

BABY'S STATS

▶ Baby's brain is getting wrinkled.

▶ Baby's hands are now fully developed

▶ Baby is grasping things.

▶ Fat cells are regulating body temperature, so lanugo is disappearing.

▶ Baby's bone marrow is now making red blood cells.

MOM'S STATS

▶ Her ligaments are beginning to relax.

▶ The urge to pee is constant.

▶ Her breasts have increased in size, and the discomfort continues.

▶ Mom's lack of sleep causes exhaustion. Essential oils like lavender might be great in an oil diffuser, but you'll need to consult with a holistic expert to make sure you're using something that isn't harmful for the developing baby. Doctors will recommend that Mom limit the amount of tea that she's consuming, so that may not be an option.

NOT-TO-MISS APPOINTMENTS

▶ Your second third-trimester appointment may be happening. Mom might be screened for staph, which could be passed to the baby through breastfeeding. A "kick count" test may be done to determine baby's health. Another potential ultrasound could be scheduled.

Family Goals

DADDY DOULA Help Mom feel good on her feet: If you managed to avoid making playful jokes about your partner's feet and are still alive, ask her if she's happy with the shoes she has—they could be a major factor in keeping her toes and arches less sore. If not, take her out for a second round of shoe shopping—in case the ones she bought earlier aren't doing the trick anymore!

HOME CEO Home safety/babyproofing: If you haven't done any research on what it takes to babyproof your house, take some of your downtime and start making a list. Tour your apartment or house and see what you can initially spot with common sense, like open electricity outlets, household cleaners below the sink, and your hidden weapons (à la Dwight Schrute on *The Office*). Then, compare your list to a professional list and realize that there are so many more hazards that can be eliminated before baby comes home.

CONVERSATION STARTERS Begin talking about a fourth-trimester plan: Sleep is extremely important for both parents once the baby is born, and it's never too early to begin talking about how the two of you will manage that process. Who will get up in the middle of the night to feed the baby? If Mom is breastfeeding and pumping, will Dad do this? If Dad works full time, will he handle weekend nights while Mom covers weekdays? Without at least four to six hours of uninterrupted sleep, both of you will be useless. If neither parent can sacrifice losing sleep or uphold tag-team duties, perhaps you should look into hiring a night nurse or doula to help with the first few weeks.

Head Turning

Even though your baby is rapidly approaching birth length and weighs about three pounds, it has another three to five pounds to gain before it makes its debut. Your baby is making a trillion brain connections and already processing information, tracking light, and perceiving signals from all five senses. It is also sleeping a lot longer these days, getting that valuable REM sleep, and Mom can definitely begin to tell the waking hours from the sleeping hours.

Mom is feeling all of those consistent discomforts, and the Braxton Hicks contractions are increasing day by day. Only she can learn and tell the difference between what might be a Braxton Hicks contraction and the *we're having a baby* version, so you've got to stay on your toes and listen to her instincts. Sciatic pain is fairly normal. It happens when the baby is punching, kicking, or resting on the sciatic nerve—which will cause a shooting pain from the back down through the legs.

Restless legs syndrome is less common (affecting maybe 15 percent of pregnant women), but it is still a real pain in the rear for those who experience it, especially at night when Mom is trying to sleep. Acupuncture, yoga, and meditation seem to

BABY'S STATS

- Baby weighs close to 3½ pounds and is the size of a coconut.
- Baby is now kicking, flipping, hiccuping, and punching the uterus.
- Baby's body fat is increasing.
- Baby can move its head side to side.

MOM'S STATS

- Mom's Braxton Hicks contractions increase in frequency and intensity.
- Mom can *really* feel baby moving, and this can even wake her up at night.
- Mom's discomforts continue.
- Mom may realize when baby is napping and want to nap at the same time.

NOT-TO-MISS APPOINTMENTS

- See Week 30.

quell the creeping burning and tingling feeling that overtakes the legs and ruins a good night of sleep.

Another top-shelf dilemma is "lightning crotch." I'll give you a minute while you clean up that spit-take of whatever you were drinking and right yourself. Lightning crotch is real. It's not a

Funny or Die parody video (yet); it's actually a vicious pain that many doctors can offer theories on but can't quite explain. It's an occasional, intense shooting pain that sends a burst of pain deep into the pelvis or vagina—described by some women as a sharp jabbing or electric shock. Some doctors have considered that this sudden stinging, burning feeling could be attributed to the baby pressing on the nerve that leads to the cervix, but it's impossible to pinpoint. So if your partner drops to her knees and shrieks in horror in the middle of a Sunday-morning church sermon and you pick her up from between the pews, just remember that she may not need an exorcism.

With the baby coming shortly, it's not a bad idea to start banking meals while you still have the energy and ambition. When Jen and I had our first two kids, we lived in an apartment in Los Angeles. We didn't have much space for anything, let alone a second refrigerator or deep freezer in the garage (part of why we moved back east). If we had had one of those available, I may have considered this option. If you're a first-time parent, you can only rely on what other people who have gone through this have told you. I'd like to join the pile-on by telling you that once the baby is born, any little tip like this will pay dividends tenfold.

Family Goals

PLAN AHEAD Meal preparation: Make a batch of homemade lasagna and divvy it up into portions, drop it into gallon-size freezer bags, and date it. Or take locally harvested basil and make pesto that you can freeze for serving later with pasta. Frozen meals will be a comfort for those days when you just can't see straight—meals made from scratch that will take only minutes to bring back to life.

BROWNIE POINTS Buy a push gift: I'm not certain when the "push gift" became a thing. I just know that all of a sudden, when my wife was entering her third trimester with our daughter, people began to ask, "What are you getting her as a gift?" My initial reply was "Isn't the baby the gift?" And I haven't bothered to eat my shoe since. It's never a bad idea to pick up a special piece of sentimental jewelry that Mom can emotionally attach to. This time around, not as a "push gift" but just as a surprise, I got my wife a silver necklace on Etsy that had four little chicks on it—one for each of our kids—and she said that it's the best thing I've ever bought her. Another time, I managed to obtain a copy of our unborn baby's heartbeat from the Doppler as a JPEG file and had it made into a silver piece of jewelry. Birthstones and initial jewelry are other great options.

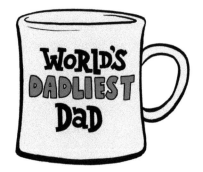

CHAPTER EIGHT

The Eighth Month

With only one more month to go after this, you and your partner are either loving every minute of it or are somewhat weary of the past several months. Either way, this beautiful bundle of joy is coming soon!

It's imperative that Mom get as much rest as possible this month, and high time that you run through the trimester checklists to make sure that you don't get caught with your pants down—that's what got you here! If you're behind on prepping your house for the baby and locking down all of the accessories that come along with being a new parent, you'll need to kick it into high gear these remaining weeks.

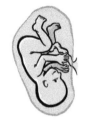

8-MONTH FETUS

NEW GEAR

opaque skin, skull

SIZE COMPARISON

Nerf football, a size 12 men's shoe

NOTES

inhales and exhales, responds to pain,
positions downward

Fully Developed Organs

This week, all of your baby's organs are completely developed, with the lungs still inhaling and exhaling amniotic fluid as baby prepares to breathe on its own. Baby is continuing to gain fat—like you and I from November through January—and its skin is finally opaque. The baby is almost 3½ to 4 pounds and as big as 15 to 17 inches.

Mom is feeling bigger and bigger. Sleep is coming in spurts, and that makes it difficult to keep an even mood and concentrate on anything. Make sure that your partner is continuing to eat small, nourishing meals and sleep with her head elevated—a way to counter heartburn.

Family Goals

DADDY DOULA Keep her moods and feet elevated: Encourage Mom to elevate her head at night and utilize the wedge or sleeping pillow to get her legs into a position that's comfortable enough for her to get some rest.

BABY'S STATS

▶ Baby weighs around four pounds and is the size of a spaghetti squash.

▶ Every organ is developed except the lungs.

▶ Baby is working on inhaling and exhaling amniotic fluid.

▶ Baby's skin is finally opaque.

MOM'S STATS

▶ Her fundal height may be between 12½ and 13½ inches, and the belly is getting bigger.

▶ Her belly button may start to resemble an outie.

▶ Baby may be dropping lower, putting more pressure on the bladder.

▶ The Braxton Hicks contractions continue to strengthen.

▶ Breast leakage and vaginal discharge are possible.

NOT-TO-MISS APPOINTMENTS

▶ Stay up-to-date on third-trimester test results. If she was tested for staph, these results should be available. They will factor into the decision on whether she'll be able to breastfeed.

PLAN AHEAD Finalize the birth plan: It's finally time to pull the trigger on a definitive birth plan that you can share with your doctor and their team. If Mom is too overwhelmed in the delivery room, you (and possibly her doula) are her biggest advocate and spokesperson. You need to be prepared to help guide the doctor into following your birth plan and be able to speak up with confidence if there are complications and you need to deviate. The one thing having children will teach you is that nothing happens on time—and rarely, if ever, according to plan. Be flexible and have a backup plan, but stick to your guns if you and your partner feel strongly about something. This is also a good time to discuss if you and your partner want to opt for cord blood banking.

Flexible Skull

Your baby is gaining about half a pound a week and is doing a lot of preparation for life outside the womb. The consistent intake of amniotic fluid is preparing its digestive system for feeding. The skull isn't fully fused yet, and there's a reason for this. The baby will need this flexibility in order to get through the birth canal. The area in which the skull isn't fully fused is known as the "fontanel" but is more commonly referred to as the "soft spot."

Mom is in the final stretches of what has been a long journey. She's tired, uncomfortable, and can't stop talking about getting this baby out of her belly. She's hungry all the time but has trouble eating because of the heartburn and discomfort.

While labor and childbirth are still a few weeks away, it's important that Mom familiarize herself with the difference between urine leakage and amniotic fluid leakage. Urine is most often yellow (you probably knew this) and has a faint or pungent smell of ammonia, while amniotic fluid is pale and clear and has a sweeter smell. I've only been privy to encountering amniotic fluid once, and it was late at night during our second pregnancy with Charlie. My wife's water had broken in bed and while it didn't wake me up at first—my wife's

BABY'S STATS

▶ Baby is gaining about half a pound a week.

▶ Baby is likely in a head-down position and dropping to the lower pelvis.

▶ Baby's skull isn't fully fused yet, as it needs that flexibility as it passes through the birth canal. This is why babies are born with a "soft spot," also known as the "fontanel."

MOM'S STATS

▶ The top of Mom's uterus is about five inches above her pubic bones right now, and her belly is round and *large*.

▶ She may be carrying the baby lower.

▶ She's most likely tired and irritable, mainly because of the discomfort, which is normal from now until the birth.

▶ She's most likely not sleeping well.

▶ Mom may often feel hungry because so many nutrients are going to the baby; but it may be difficult for her to eat because eating often causes discomfort and heartburn.

NOT-TO-MISS APPOINTMENTS

▶ See Week 30.

▶ Confirm that you're registered with the hospital or birthing center.

punching me in the back did—she told me that it almost made the sound of a water balloon being popped softly. She was never sure if it actually made a sound that I could hear or if she could hear it inside her own body, but she certainly felt it as it happened. That's when I flew into panic mode . . . but I'll save that for a bit later in the book.

Family Goals

DAD RD Make her something easy to eat: It might be tough for Mom to stomach a lot of meals, whether because of nausea or smell. In order to combat this, I came up with a protein smoothie that gave my wife the nutrients that both she *and* the baby needed.

PLAN AHEAD Tour the hospital or birthing center: My wife and I toured each of the hospitals that she gave birth in. Almost all hospitals and birthing centers offer parents the opportunity to come in and walk through the labor and delivery units and postpartum recovery rooms. You can become familiar with the sights and sounds of the hospital, and it's definitely not a bad idea to do a dry run. This helps you get an idea of where the emergency room is, where to park, whether you'll need to stop and grab a parking ticket (instead of gunning it through the guard gates like a wild first-time dad on a rampage), and what constitutes the general layout of the facility and its rules and processes so you can share that information with your family, in-laws, and friends.

CONVERSATION STARTERS Discuss who you want at the hospital and in the delivery room: My wife and I are of the mind-set "the more the merrier" in the hospital waiting room and for visitors during postpartum care in the hospital. We think of this as our baby's very first birthday party. We invite all of our families and very close friends to be there. But as much as we wanted everyone with us to celebrate our baby's arrival, we didn't want anyone else in the delivery room. That was for us, a private moment to share together, and each couple needs to make these decisions on their own. That said, some couples decide that they want their mothers and mothers-in-law (or other special family members such as godparents) to be present for the delivery. This is an important conversation to have as a couple to make sure you are on the same page about expectations for privacy. Additionally, all hospitals have guidelines about the number of people allowed in delivery rooms, and some have rules about the number of people at any given time who can visit during postpartum. (Also, it never hurts to bribe your nurses—a dozen donuts here, a bucket of candy there—and you can pretty much sweet-talk your way into being the favorite patient in the wing.)

Vernix

Your baby is 17 to 18 inches long and almost five pounds this week. For Mom, it's almost like carrying around a bag of granulated sugar with limbs. If it's a boy, those testicles have almost completed their rappel from the abdomen down into the scrotum. Keep in mind, about 3 to 4 percent of boys are born without descended testicles. Don't sweat it; in most cases, they drop before the boy's first birthday. And if they don't, again there's nothing to worry about. Trust me, I've gone through this. Just consult your pediatrician, and they'll refer you to a specialist.

Another cool thing that happened is your baby's fingernails have finally reached the tips of its fingers. It's always good to add buying a fingernail clipper (unless you're old-school and use baby nail scissors) to your to-do checklist. They make them with safety guards in the event that you get a little ambitious and clip them too short. A word of advice: Clip or trim them while baby is sleeping; it might end up being a little less aggressive of a situation.

Mom is hanging in there. As I mentioned previously, think about carrying around a sack of sugar in your stomach and issue sympathy accordingly. Mom's uterus is anywhere from 500 to 1,000 times bigger than when we started this journey.

BABY'S STATS

▶ Baby is about five pounds and the size of a cantaloupe. Its head is likely down and dropping toward the pelvis.

▶ Baby's fingernails reach the fingertips now.

▶ Baby's lungs are in the final week of development.

▶ If it's a boy, the testicles have fully descended.

MOM'S STATS

▶ Mom's uterus is taking up significant room and causing discomfort.

▶ She may be experiencing some anxiety related to the whole idea of childbirth.

▶ She's tired and urinating *a lot*.

▶ Increased urinary output may have Mom feeling tired of drinking fluids, but the reality is that she needs to stay hydrated.

NOT-TO-MISS APPOINTMENTS

▶ Do at least one dry run to the hospital to make sure you know the route and alternate routes. The weekend before a planned C-section for our second child's birth, a major highway system closure in Los Angeles caused a traffic jam that became known as "Carmageddon." Almost nothing about having children happens on your schedule, so it wasn't really a surprise when my wife's water broke that Sunday and we found ourselves taking back roads to get to the hospital, which took us twice as long.

She hasn't been able to see below her waist in weeks and has to lie on her back just to make sure that her shoes are on the right feet. She's stressed out, as many moms are leading up to the delivery. She's most likely full of anxiety about what will happen in the next few weeks since women have been sharing their birth stories with her ever since the two of you announced the pregnancy. That stuff gets inside of your head. Do everything you can to make her comfortable and relieve the stress.

Family Goals

DADDY DOULA Be the waterboy: Much like my old friend the original waterboy, Bobby Boucher Jr. (played by Adam Sandler), would say, "No, no, you people are drinking the wrong water." Forget about caffeinated drinks or anything with artificial coloring or flavors. H_2O is where it's at. Mom needs to drink her water, and a lot of it. Maybe you could cruise Amazon Prime for a new water bottle in her favorite color for a surprise. S'well and CamelBak make great options!

PLAN AHEAD Install your car seat: Back in the day, you used to be able to pull into a fire station and have a firefighter install your seat for you, but alas, I believe those days are over. It's going to take some time to figure out how to do the install. Consult your vehicle handbook for the approved process, and pull up some YouTube videos on installing your particular brand, just to be extra sure.

A Big Milestone

This week is huge. Your baby has lungs that are now fully developed. If born now, baby has a good chance of breathing on their own, which is amazing! The kidneys and liver are fully developed, as are all other organs. Baby is about 18 inches and a little over five pounds. The rest of the ride is spent gaining a bit of weight and building up that big old brain. If it hasn't happened already, the baby is likely flipping head down to get ready for delivery.

If the baby hasn't made the move south yet, Mom may have moments in which she's short of breath. Her Braxton Hicks contractions are continuing to make an appearance and it's very easy to mistake them for the real deal. She's most likely tired from going through normal daily motions, and it's time (if you haven't done so already) for Dad to step up and take care of business around the house. I'm somewhat obsessive, but I like to try and stay one step ahead of my wife. I take a few minutes to remove the 40 decorative pillows (don't get me started) from our bed, fill up her essential oil diffuser (with pregnancy-safe oils, check on that!), and make sure she has water on deck before she even gets into the room. And I don't do it just on Thursday, Sunday, and Monday nights when

BABY'S STATS

▶ Baby is the size of a small Nerf football.

▶ Baby's lungs are fully developed.

▶ Baby's kidneys and liver, as well as all other organs, are fully developed.

▶ Baby is just putting on weight.

MOM'S STATS

▶ If the baby hasn't dropped yet, it's putting a lot of pressure on Mom's lungs, which may lead to shortness of breath.

▶ If the baby is dropping, Mom will notice some relief of those symptoms, but on the flip side, the baby is now pressing more exclusively on the bladder.

▶ Her Braxton Hicks contractions are increasing in frequency, and it's easy to mistake them for the *real thing*.

NOT-TO-MISS APPOINTMENTS

▶ This is the last week of appointments being every two weeks; baby can come at any time now.

football is on . . . wink, wink. But if I can manage to get the kids in bed and my wife settled so that I can watch a few snaps uninterrupted, am I going to hell? No, and you won't either.

Family Goals

HOME CEO Take over around the house: Whatever daily household maintenance you can get to before she does is a win. Whether it is taking the pets out to go to the bathroom, making dinner or cleaning up the kitchen, or getting laundry going, do what you can so Mom can kick her feet up and get that much-needed rest.

PLAN AHEAD Pack a bag: Dude, this is a final warning. Our second and third babies came early, and I had procrastinated. I ended up throwing my bag together as my wife was cleaning amniotic fluid off of our duvet (don't ask). Let's just say that my hospital wardrobe was a combination of wrinkled dress shirts and swim trunks. This is a warning: Don't be like me.

PLAN AHEAD Labor and delivery plan: We're not talking about a birth plan—you should've already nailed that and be on the same page with your partner and the doctor. I'm talking about who is going to feed the fish and turn on a few lights at night so that you don't get robbed.

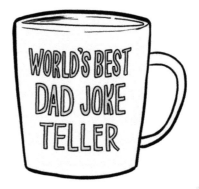

CHAPTER NINE

The Ninth Month

It's been a long road, but you're finally here. This is the month that everyone's been waiting for . . . unless of course, you don't deliver until month 10, in which case hang in there!

Mom is most likely tired, uncomfortable in every position, and can't wait to sleep on her stomach *and* see her feet and her vagina once again. Baby is continuing to gain weight and hopefully getting into a position to be born.

This month seems like it takes forever to go by, but you'll be able to keep yourself busy with last-minute preparations to the nursery and apartment, or house, and with finishing up projects at work in the event you need to rush to the hospital at any given moment. There will most likely be no shortage of family and friends reaching out to you to get your address, ask which hospital you'll be at, and share any other details that pop into their heads. Don't get so caught up with everything on the periphery that you don't take some time to enjoy quiet time with your partner and the moment that is bringing a new smiling face into this world!

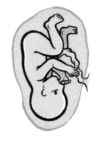

9-MONTH FETUS

NEW GEAR

vocal cords, fully developed lungs, kidneys,
intestines, rapid brain development

SIZE COMPARISON

watermelon, large movie popcorn, chihuahua

NOTES

hears, blinks, grasps

In the Homestretch

Your baby is weighing in around six pounds and probably measuring 18 to 19 inches in length. Congratulations, you're in the homestretch. For those of you who have ever smoked a brisket using the traditional method—choosing your wood carefully, checking in on and monitoring the process, maintaining that steady heat for hours and hours on end—that process is not that far from what you are experiencing right now. Caring for and showing that brisket some tender loving care, then taking it off the smoker and letting it rest is like watching your baby being born and seeing them fall asleep on their mother's chest. There's such a comfort and joy that overwhelms you.

Okay, okay . . . maybe I've pushed my analogies to an uncomfortably meaty level, but I'm about to have a fourth child—and it's the simple things that commandeer my emotions, people. The circulatory and musculoskeletal systems are ready to rock. The digestive system is ready, too, but it hasn't gotten a workout yet. But hang onto your butts—literally. It's coming.

BABY'S STATS

▶ Baby is fully developed and continues to gain weight.

▶ Baby is the size of a head of romaine lettuce.

▶ Baby's movements in the womb are more subtle now.

▶ Baby's cheeks are filling out.

▶ Baby is forming meconium from swallowing amniotic fluid.

MOM'S STATS

▶ Hormones are loosening Mom's connective tissue in preparation for delivery.

▶ Lightening (the baby dropping lower) may still be happening.

▶ She has swelling in her lower extremities, back pain, and poor sleep that can cause irritability.

NOT-TO-MISS APPOINTMENTS

▶ Appointments are now down to once a week. The doctor will be checking the position of the baby and the height of the uterus, and continuing to monitor urine, weight, and blood pressure. Mom may need an ultrasound to determine the position of the baby. If your schedule allows, it would be ideal if you could make these weekly visits.

Family Goals

HOME CEO Let her kick her feet up: Continue with the practice of staying one step ahead of her at home by pulling as many duties as you can. You have no idea how much of a relief it will be for your partner.

DADDY DOULA Naptime for Mom: Do whatever you can to encourage Mom to get rest when she can, even if it's at the expense of missing friendly get-togethers or work-related events. Those people will understand. And if they don't, they probably haven't gone through this process themselves.

Early Term

The exciting news this week is that if your baby is born, he will be considered either "at term" or "full term" and is no longer premature. Note: Only about 5 percent of babies arrive on their actual due date and about 6.4 percent are born at 37 weeks. This is more likely with multiples. The baby continues to gain weight at around a half pound per week, and the average fetus weighs around 6½ pounds, although weight does vary from fetus to fetus as it does from newborn to newborn. Fat continues to accumulate, and the baby is still inhaling and exhaling amniotic fluid and flipping from side to side in the womb.

Mom could experience a surge of energy as you come close to birth, and if you haven't been paying attention around the house, there's most likely been some nesting going on. It's a natural instinct to want to organize and clean things up around you and offer the best possible scenario for your baby to enter the world.

Does this mean that it might be a pain in the ass from time to time? Yes. Will you find yourself mumbling curse words on occasion as you move furniture around the house as if it's a game of musical chairs on steroids? Yes. Will you don a fake smile and wave excitedly to your partner from the front yard

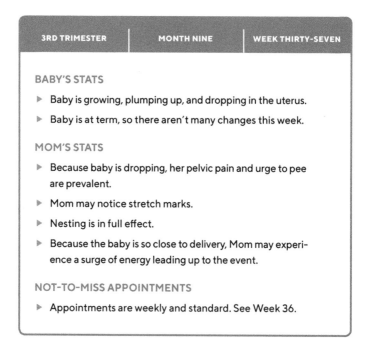

BABY'S STATS

▶ Baby is growing, plumping up, and dropping in the uterus.

▶ Baby is at term, so there aren't many changes this week.

MOM'S STATS

▶ Because baby is dropping, her pelvic pain and urge to pee are prevalent.

▶ Mom may notice stretch marks.

▶ Nesting is in full effect.

▶ Because the baby is so close to delivery, Mom may experience a surge of energy leading up to the event.

NOT-TO-MISS APPOINTMENTS

▶ Appointments are weekly and standard. See Week 36.

as you power wash the siding on the house while missing the Masters Tournament? Of course, but smile and work on your gratitude. Bringing a child into this world is one of the most amazing things you'll ever do in your life.

Family Goals

PLAN AHEAD Review the action plan: This is it. This is go time. Everyone is on high alert. This isn't the time to accidentally leave your cell phone in a friend's car. If you're worried about that happening, swallow your pride, take one for the team, and get a fancy hip clip holster. Stay in daily contact with everyone who's included in your emergency plan. Keep in touch, even if it's just a quick update on how Mom is feeling.

DAD RD Be the meal warden: Encourage your partner, as difficult as it may be, to eat small meals or snacks at various times throughout the day. The nutrition will keep her strength up and also continue to bulk up that little baby you've got coming.

Ready to Meet You

Your baby is now clocking in at seven pounds and measuring near the 20-inch mark. Even though there could potentially be another two weeks (four at the max) in utero, your baby is ready to hit the ground running, which means crying. It is still in the process of shedding the vernix, the greasy white substance that protects its skin. Everything else is ready to go; baby is simply gaining weight and allowing the wisdom of Mother Nature to decide when it's time.

Mom is experiencing the baby dropping into the pelvis, and her cervix may be softening and may have even begun dilating at this point. Her appetite probably isn't the best—it's difficult to eat any kind of large meal because there's no space to put it! Healthy protein shakes or bars are an excellent choice. The baby is taking up so much room that it almost becomes frustrating. Mom is continuing to have feelings of anxiety and hope about having a successful delivery and moving on to the next step—bringing baby home.

Unless you have a scheduled C-section, it's always a gamble when Mom decides to begin her maternity leave. If it's a natural birth, most couples want to get that extra week of work and pay logged to help them out financially; however, you don't want to

BABY'S STATS

▶ Baby is fully developed and continues to add weight.

▶ Baby weighs about 7½ pounds and is almost as long as a football.

▶ Baby's toenails now reach the end of the toes.

▶ Baby's vocal cords are fully developed.

MOM'S STATS

▶ Baby is continuing to drop in the pelvis, and Mom's cervix is softening and dilating.

▶ Her nesting continues.

▶ Anywhere you go, Mom has already scoped out the bathroom.

NOT-TO-MISS APPOINTMENTS

▶ There are appointments every week. If the baby is breech, the doctor will have already scheduled or is in the process of scheduling a C-section.

compromise the front end of your birth plan, which is getting to the hospital in the safest and least stressful way possible. You're rolling the dice on this one, and the barometer should be how Mom feels about her body.

Family Goals

☑ PLAN AHEAD Start maternity leave: Obviously, everyone at Mom's work knows that she's almost done with this pregnancy, and if she's still working, she may want to consult with her employer and consider taking maternity leave now so she can rest at home and relieve some worry that she might go into labor on the job.

☑ PLAN AHEAD Request paternity leave: If you're lucky enough to work for a company that offers this, you'll have to plan carefully, as you'll want to take advantage of every day available to you. Hopefully, your employer will be in tune with your situation and be comfortable if you've got to run out in the middle of the day. An even better scenario is if her mother or another family member is able to spend time with Mom in the week or two leading up to the due date so you can save your paternity leave dates for the postpartum trenches. Note: C-sections are a lot easier to plan for, as you have a relatively set date for delivery.

WHEN A C-SECTION IS NECESSARY

A C-section birth is the surgical delivery of an infant through incisions made in the mother's abdomen and uterus. There are many reasons that a C-section might be necessary, but one of the most common is when the baby is in a breech position. Breech position is when the baby fails to maneuver its head toward the birth canal and instead, sits in an upright position. Recovery times are extended for a C-section, and your hospital stay will be a bit longer. A C-section will also result in a more complex healing process.

Any Day Now

Your baby weighs in at between seven and eight pounds, measures between 19 and 21 inches, and has essentially stopped growing until delivery. The brain development hasn't stopped, and that continues for the first few years. The old skin is sloughing off, and new skin is taking its place. Baby is no longer pink in color but rather a white or whitish-gray that will ultimately change its pigmentation upon arrival.

Mom may be frustrated by now, wishing that the baby would finally come. The anxiety of the unknown is there, as well as the discomfort that ultimately causes irritability. Now is a great time to work on finishing up your to-do list, including the nursery, hospital bag, and cleaning and organizing around the house.

Family Goals

DADDY DOULA Promote self-care: Mom needs to take care of herself during this critical time. Warm baths are a great thing, as well as plenty of rest and continuing to eat small meals. Mom should keep her feet up and not do too much in the way of household maintenance or work. Encourage Mom to read a new book or catch up on Netflix.

BABY'S STATS

▶ Baby is close to birth weight and forming new skin as old skin sloughs off.

▶ Baby probably weighs between seven and eight pounds and is continuing to fill out.

▶ Baby is the size of a mini-watermelon and full term.

MOM'S STATS

▶ Baby's position may pinch nerves and, as a result, cause more occurrences of that wonderful lightning crotch.

▶ All her previous discomforts continue. With the baby continuing to grow, sleep will be tough, eating will be a chore, and moving around doing day-to-day activities will be slow going.

NOT-TO-MISS APPOINTMENTS

▶ The weekly check-in appointments continue.

PREGNANCY EMPATHY 101 Be on call: If the baby hasn't arrived yet, Mom is most likely mentally exhausted and physically unable to do much of anything. It kind of feels as if you're both sitting around . . . waiting. The best thing you can do is to ensure that she's comfortable and has everything she needs without having to go out of her way.

Finally!

Congratulations, you've reached the end of your pregnancy!
Your baby weighs between six and nine pounds and measures
between 19 and 22 inches, though healthy babies clock in anywhere on either end of that spectrum. About 30 percent of all
babies are born during this week, but yours may want to stay in
a bit longer, which is totally fine. Your practitioner most likely
won't allow Mom to go over 42 weeks.

Mom is absolutely huge and ready for this to happen. Her
cervix is softening and starting to dilate. She's most likely
experiencing discomfort and is excited, terrified, nervous,
sleep deprived, and anything else that you can think of. She
could really use your support in every way possible—physical,
mental, and emotional.

Family Goals

DADDY DOULA Be the rock: Provide reassurance
to your partner that you're going to be with her
100 percent of the way. You're the point person—you're
the contact for anyone involved in your birth plan, anyone
visiting from out of town, and those who couldn't make it

BABY'S STATS

▶ Baby is at whatever the birth weight will be. The doctor can guess, but more than likely you won't know until they put the baby on the scale.

MOM'S STATS

▶ Baby has dropped and is in position for birth.

▶ Mom's cervix continues to soften and dilate.

▶ Mom is probably uncomfortable, excited, terrified, nervous, and sleep deprived. She is also anxious about beginning her life as a mom.

▶ Mom won't be getting her period for several more weeks.

▶ If it's go time for Mom, keep in mind that she will deliver not only a baby but also the placenta (often referred to as the second birth).

NOT-TO-MISS APPOINTMENTS

▶ The weekly appointments continue; the doctor may discuss inducing labor.

and want updates or FaceTime chats to wish Mom well. Arm yourself with parking information at the hospital, the floor number, and the recovery room that you're in. People will need this information to send food or flowers . . . Hopefully, no strip-o-grams.

HOME CEO One final cleanup: If the baby hasn't arrived yet and you're both sitting around waiting, it might be a good time to clean the apartment or house one final time before you bring the baby home. There's nothing worse than coming home from the hospital with a new baby and finding a mess.

DAD RD Induce labor through food: You can also score brownie points with this one. Almost every city across the country has a fabled restaurant . . . You know, *that* place where women are rumored to go into labor from eating a specific dish. In the San Fernando Valley, it's known as Caioti Pizza Cafe, and "The Salad" is rumored to kick women's bodies into labor within 24 hours. Be the hero and check out some local blogs to see if there is a rumored place where you can take your partner.

Will There Ever Be a Baby?

Your baby is coming; don't fret. Around 15 to 20 percent of babies are born in weeks 41 and 42, and if not, the doctor will normally induce labor or talk to you about the C-section option. The baby is full-term and continues developing its brain functions.

All of our babies were born prior to 40 weeks, so I don't necessarily know the mental struggle that couples endure at this point. I can only equate it to how I felt during weeks 36, 37, and 38. As a husband and father, I had a lot of anxiety. I wasn't sure when I was going to "get the call" and treated my cell phone like it was the Holy Grail. I would continue to check and make sure I had 100 percent battery life, that I was always in zones with three and four bars, and if anyone called me "just to chat," I hurried my conversation and got off the call almost immediately. I didn't care about how Steve got hammered at the bar, forgot where he parked, and had to take an Uber to work. I was laser focused on one thing.

BABY'S STATS

▶ About 16 percent of babies are born in Week 41 and another 1 percent during Week 42.

▶ Baby isn't considered post-term until 42 weeks, and the doctor will more than likely induce or deliver via C-section before that time comes.

▶ Baby is full-term and continues to add fat.

MOM'S STATS

▶ The Week 40 changes are still in effect.

▶ She might be having difficulty wrapping her head around missing the due date, which could create a bit of a letdown.

▶ Her anxiety is running full tilt.

NOT-TO-MISS APPOINTMENTS

▶ Weekly appointments are still happening, and induction or C-section are being discussed.

Family Goals

 PLAN AHEAD Keep your hospital bags handy: As we got to this point in the pregnancy, I always took my hospital bag with me to work and brought it home every night. It lived by the front door, just in case.

 PLAN AHEAD Talk through your classes: If you happened to take Lamaze or other childbirth classes, take 15 minutes each night to practice breathing with your partner. This will help keep the techniques fresh in both of your minds.

 DADDY DOULA Take care of Dad: Self-care is still of the utmost importance. Take a moment to meditate or go on a quick run to keep you sane.

THE THIRD-TRIMESTER CHECKLIST

HOME:

- ☐ Babyproof your home.
- ☐ Install the car seat.
- ☐ Make sure that you have your hospital bag with you at all times. Make sure your partner's bag is packed and by the front door or accessible at all times.
- ☐ Help your partner write out thank-you cards for baby gifts.
- ☐ Start making meals that you can store in the freezer.

BABY:

- ☐ Talk with your partner about what you are looking for in a pediatrician. Gather referrals, research online, and interview potential candidates.
- ☐ Enroll in childcare and infant/child CPR classes.
- ☐ Practice what you learn in the classes with your partner. It will help you keep the techniques fresh in both of your minds.

MOM:

- ☐ Practice what you learned at childbirth and Lamaze classes.
- ☐ Establish a sleep plan with Mom for when the baby comes and how you and your partner will manage night-time feedings and changings.
- ☐ Consider giving a sentimental push gift for your partner.

PRENATAL APPOINTMENTS:

☐ Checkup appointments will be every two weeks starting at Week 28 and then switch to once a week starting at Week 36 until labor.

☐ Mom will be tested for Group B Strep.

HOSPITAL:

☐ Finalize the birth plan with your partner, your doula (if you hired one), and the obstetrician.

☐ Tour the hospital or birthing center.

☐ Have the action plan ready to go for when your partner goes into labor.

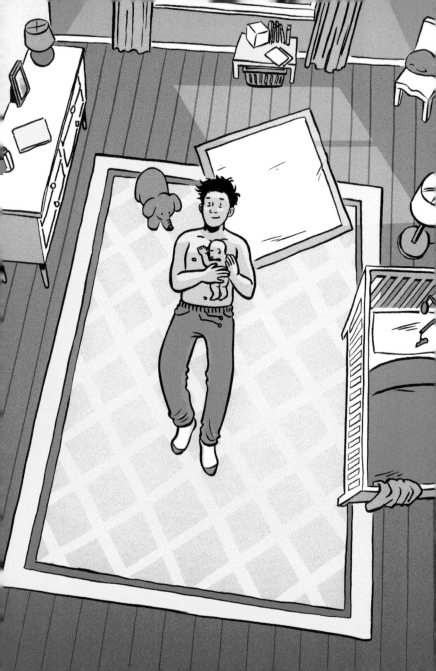

PART FOUR

THE "FOURTH TRIMESTER"

A final round of congratulations is in order—welcome to the club, Dad! A lot of people don't think about the fact that Mom needs a good 40 days to recover from the entire process. It takes another several weeks for both parents and baby to get on any type of routine or schedule. That's one of the reasons why we think that the three months after delivery deserves its own designation as a trimester.

If you're reading this, you've hopefully survived your stay at the hospital and managed to somehow white-knuckle it home on your maiden voyage with precious cargo in the back seat. I'll never forget my virgin ride from the hospital to our apartment. I was hugging the right lane doing 35 mph, screaming at every other maniac on the road—didn't they know that I was transporting a newborn?!

Once you're home, most couples don't do much during that first week or two—simply make sure that all of the baby's needs are met. And if your parents or in-laws aren't around to give a hand, it's up to Dad to step up and stay on top of all of the household duties, as well as make sure that Mom is not doing *anything* she doesn't need to do . . . other than rest and breastfeed. After a few weeks, those routines and schedules will define themselves, and it's important to get those set before people start going back to work.

And while all this is happening, the most important part of this "fourth trimester" is to spend quality time with this gorgeous, beautiful baby that you created together. Enjoy an abundance of quiet time looking into baby's eyes, allowing the baby skin-to-skin contact on Dad's chest, and letting him or her learn your voice, your smell, and your laugh. Before too long, you'll have your own way of communicating without even talking.

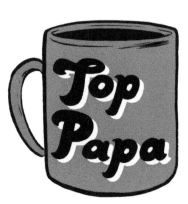

CHAPTER TEN

The Tenth Month

A majority of parents have already given birth by this time, and if you haven't, don't worry—your time is coming. For those who have, you've made it through labor and delivery (or a C-section) and triumphed over your hospital stay and nights of barely getting any sleep in a cot with worn-out mattress springs.

The next month is about doing anything and everything you can to help Mom recover, whether it is taking over household duties, pet detail, bill payment, or midnight feedings. This is a time to work with your partner and support one another so that you both get enough sleep to function. Encourage Mom to keep eating healthy, especially if she's breastfeeding. But beyond everything, this is also a time to bond with your little one . . .

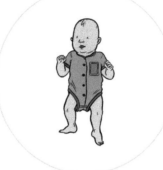

1-MONTH INFANT

AVERAGE SIZE

7 pounds

WEIGHT COMPARISON

bag of sugar, a brick

NOTES

normal weight loss first week, communicates
through cries, feeding times will get longer and
more frequent, umbilical cord will dry out and
fall out, facial expressions like smiling

Lots of Sleep for Baby, Less for You

Finally, the wait is over and your beautiful child is now here. The baby is going to lose a bit of weight during this first week, and you shouldn't be worried. You're going to begin to understand the needs of your child based on cries. It's usually one of a few things—they're either hungry, tired, have peed or pooped and need a diaper change, or just want the security of being held. The baby will have a small plastic clip that was used to clamp off the umbilical cord, and you'll need to exercise caution during diaper changes—it can be somewhat painful for the baby until it dries out and naturally falls off in the next few days. I'll spare you the story of how, with our first, the umbilical cord stump fell off and we didn't realize it until we saw the dog frantically sniffing and digging at the corner of our sofa . . .

If you chose to have your baby boy circumcised, the incision will also be healing, and you'll receive special instructions on how to care for that. You'll likely be given this option during your recovery stay, or (based on your OB/GYN's preference) you may be directed to go to an independent specialist during his first couple of weeks.

BABY'S STATS

▶ Baby will likely lose a bit of weight—about 5 percent—this week. Don't fret—this is normal.

▶ Baby will learn to latch on to Mom's breast to begin feeding.

▶ Baby will expel meconium, which is essentially black tar-like poop. Don't worry—this is also normal.

▶ The umbilical cord will likely start to dry out. In one to two weeks, it will fall off for you, like a creep, to keep in your baby book.

MOM'S STATS

▶ Mom's hormones are changing during postpartum.

▶ Her breasts are filled with milk and may be tender. If nursing, she may be experiencing sore or chapped nipples.

▶ She may be experiencing discharge from the birth, called "lochia," that is similar to a heavy period.

▶ About 80 percent of moms experience post-delivery blues—a lot of up-and-down emotions may be happening.

NOT-TO-MISS APPOINTMENTS

▶ Baby will need a checkup within the first week. Your pediatrician will likely visit you during your recovery in the hospital and do a quick visit with the baby and give instructions on when to come into their office for your first real appointment.

▶ If baby is having trouble latching, you may want to schedule an appointment with a breastfeeding consultant.

I always took it upon myself—mainly because Mom was tired and resting but also because I wanted to—to lead the charge on the first diaper change. It's a huge moment for Dad and the baby to connect, and with a nurse standing by, dads can get a good feel for how the process should be done. Trust me, get someone to take a picture, because in 18 years when they're graduating from high school and going on to college, it's a memory you'll cherish. If you didn't cover this in childbirth class or skipped it altogether, many hospitals will offer a swaddling course, as well as basic instructional information on things like changing diapers and cradling.

Your stay in the hospital varies between two and four days based on recovery time after a natural birth or C-section. I chose to never leave my wife alone in the room, and simultaneously we chose never to allow our babies to leave our sight. Many hospitals have minimized nurseries and support "rooming in" as their preferred postpartum recovery method. But generally speaking, this is your option, and you and your partner should do what you feel is best for your baby, and for both of you. Once our family members and friends started making daily trips to see the baby at the hospital, I used that time to step out to get us food and take care of other things. But each night I slept alongside my wife on a cot as nurses checked on her regularly and gave us updates on the baby. They offered to keep the baby in the nursery for a few hours so that we could both sleep for a bit, and a couple of times we took them up on this option and timed it with baby's bath or blood work. I showered there and used that hospital bag we have been talking about for the last several chapters.

Mom's hormones are in the process of changing a lot during this first week of postpartum life. Likewise, her body is recovering from birth (or surgery) at the same time she's caring for a newborn. Her breasts are now full of milk and tender. She may be trying to get the baby to latch on to her breast and begin breastfeeding. Normally the hospital or birthing center has a lactation consultant on staff who will help Mom through the initial process. This process can be physically and emotionally challenging if the baby isn't able to latch on. It's important to encourage Mom to continue trying and not throw in the towel so early. Breastfeeding is beneficial in so many ways, not just for the nurturing and bonding time but also because the milk Mom is making will provide important antibodies that will strengthen the baby's immune system. On an unrelated note, Mom will also be experiencing heavy discharge (similar to her period) called "lochia."

You'll most likely have a lot of family and close friends visiting you while you're at the hospital; everyone else will probably give you a bit of space and stop by to see you at home once you're settled. It's important to be vigilant about making sure that all of your visitors wash their hands and sanitize before holding the baby. If Mom is breastfeeding, the little one is already building a super-robust immune system by taking in breast milk with immunities from Mom.

Family Goals

DADDY DAYCARE Use those childcare skills: After baby is done feeding, he or she will most likely need to be changed—that's just how it works. Offer to do the diaper changing and practice your swaddling technique, which will help the baby feel safe, comforted, and ready to nap. If you didn't receive swaddling instructions at the hospital, there are plenty of diagrams and how-to videos online.

DADDY DAYCARE Be the primary homemaker while Mom and baby rest: Do your best to eliminate anything that your partner needs to do while she recovers and bonds with baby.

DADDY DOULA Help Mom with breastfeeding: There are a few things that you can do to assist Mom in having a better experience with this if she's having difficulty. If she's already consulted a lactation specialist, then she (and potentially you too if you went with her) is probably already educated on latching techniques, types of equipment for pumping, and how to safely store expressed breast milk. Things *you* can help with are low milk production (encourage her to nurse every time baby is hungry), excessive time with a pacifier (this decreases feeding time), and cracked or chafed nipples (buy her plenty cream for them)! Dad tip: Cabbage leaves and cold compresses work wonders for swollen and engorged breasts, but there is a side effect—lessening of milk supply—so be careful how often (or if at all) you use this technique.

DADDY DOULA Prioritize sleep above everything else: To say that you're going to be sleep deprived for a few weeks is an understatement. Ideally, Mom (and Dad) should sleep when baby sleeps. When the little one knocks out after several tries of swaddling and rocking, it might be tempting to turn on the TV, check social media, play that last round of Candy Crush, or wash the mounds of dishes piling up, but resist the urge, especially if your sleep debt is high. When it comes to night feedings, refer back to the plan that you both made about who will sleep when and who will feed the baby and change diapers while the other one gets some much-needed rest.

Growth

The baby is now feeding a lot more, and more frequently as well. Baby will more than likely get close to regaining that small amount of weight lost at birth. It's also common for your baby to begin tracking movements—so don't be surprised if they follow you across the room with their eyes!

Mom's breasts are large if she's breastfeeding, and she's still very sleep deprived. She's probably experiencing a bit of what people call the "baby blues," which is fairly normal as the hormones begin to even out. Her uterus is shrinking, although it is still enlarged from its prepregnancy size. If Mom is nursing, she may notice quicker weight loss. And during breastfeeding times, Mom tends to be hungrier and thirstier, as the body requires lot of energy to feed a hungry newborn. My wife wouldn't even sit down to nurse without a glass of water in front of her. Get ahead of that and grab a 24-pack of water bottles so you can make it easy on your partner. She may be stressed about parenting in general or about trying to resume a normal life. Now is a time to openly communicate about worries or stressors and figure out how you can work together to lessen the impact. Mom needs to continue eating a nutritious diet, as it is essential to the baby's

BABY'S STATS

▶ Baby will begin gaining back weight and may return to their birth weight.

▶ Baby will be much hungrier this week, and feeding times will be longer and more frequent.

▶ Baby is more focused and their movements are more controlled.

MOM'S STATS

▶ If she is breastfeeding, Mom's breasts are large, and her nipples are likely tender.

▶ Mom is sleep deprived and experiencing baby blues as hormones begin evening out.

▶ Her uterus is shrinking, although it's still enlarged from its prepregnancy size.

▶ If she's nursing, her weight loss will be more obvious.

▶ Nursing moms tend to be hungry and thirsty, as their bodies require lots of energy to feed a ravenous newborn.

NOT-TO-MISS APPOINTMENTS

▶ If there weren't any complications, there won't be a need for appointments.

diet, too. Everything that Mom eats or drinks reflects directly in the breast milk that the baby is getting.

Hopefully, you were able to take off of work (or maybe you're already a stay-at-home dad) this week and spend some time with Mom and baby. If not, plan on stepping in at night so that Mom can rest.

POSTPARTUM MOOD DISORDERS

Everyone expects that Mom is going to be joyous and exuberant during those first few days and weeks after giving birth, but that's simply not always the case. Mom's hormones are beginning to even out, which is often called "baby blues." To a certain degree, this is normal; however, it's important that Dad pay close attention and be able to step in if it seems like this is crossing the line into a postpartum mood disorder. Note: Postpartum Support International is a great resource for anything that has to do with pregnancy and postpartum mood disorders. They even have a section specfically for dads and partners: http://www.postpartum.net/family/tips-for-postpartum-dads-and-partners/

On that note, it's important to recognize that dads experience postpartum mood disorders, too. With the huge changes that a baby ushers into his life as well as lack of sleep and high stress levels, Dad is also susceptible. Since Mom will be too busy recovering and bonding with the baby, enlist a family member or close friend to check on you during postpartum. The Resources section (page 272) has some places that offer support.

Family Goals

FUN PROJECTS Be a historian: Chronicle your baby's growth with weekly photos (as if you weren't doing that already). My wife and I buy journals for each child and write in them every so often, as well as when huge things begin to happen in their development.

HOME CEO Be prepared for visitors: If this is your first week at home, you should prepare for the onslaught of visitors who will want to come by, drop off a gift, see the baby, and give you a big hug. You should keep in mind that anyone coming in off the streets needs to wash and disinfect! Invest in a case of Purell.

DADDY DAYCARE Play with this beautiful baby: It's so easy to just go through the motions—sleep, eat, poop—but don't forget to play. This is one of the greatest bonding moments with baby. Sing, dance, and try and get a reaction from them with toys that make sound.

POSTPARTUM EMPATHY 101 Help alleviate Mom's labor pains and recover: As you probably witnessed, labor is painful as hell, and it doesn't end when the baby is born. Mom has likely endured some tearing (and possibly stitches) during vaginal birth, and for women who had C-sections, the stiches are new and not even close to being healed. Be extra supportive by preparing ice packs, fetching things when needed, and simply making sure she isn't overexerting herself. Additionally, the shrinking of the uterus, which happens both naturally over time and is also triggered with the start of a nursing session, can be a somewhat uncomfortable process—especially if Mom has had a C-section. If she seems to be in pain, speak to her OB/GYN or care provider about what over-the-counter (OTC) pain medication she can take. Even though the baby isn't in utero anymore, many medications pass through the breast milk, so make sure everything your partner takes—including vitamins, supplements, and OTC medications—is approved by the doctor first.

Getting to Know You

Your baby is gaining between five and seven ounces a week and is starting to use their eyes to focus on more complex shapes. Baby is sleeping between 15 and 17 hours a day, broken up in between feedings. Their digestive system is working a lot harder now, and you may notice an excess of gas and spitting up.

Mom's uterus is still shrinking, and she may be losing weight. There's still no green light on exercise or sexual intercourse. She may be experiencing bouts of incontinence, as her muscles may have weakened during the labor and delivery process. Her breasts may be sore and her nipples may be chapped.

This is most likely your second week at home with the baby and is a perfect time to begin finding your footing on a family schedule, especially if you have to go back to work. Getting into a routine at home will help both you and your partner relieve a bit of stress.

BABY'S STATS

▶ Baby is gaining about five to seven ounces per week.

▶ The digestive system is kicking into gear.

▶ The umbilical cord will likely be dry enough to fall off.

▶ Baby's eyes are focusing on more complex shapes now.

▶ Baby is sleeping an average of 15 to 17 hours per day, but not all at one time.

MOM'S STATS

▶ Her uterus is shrinking, and Mom is losing weight.

▶ It's still not safe for Mom to exercise or have sexual intercourse for a few weeks yet.

▶ Her abdominal muscles are still stretched, so she may still look somewhat pregnant.

▶ She may have incontinence from weakened muscles due to labor and delivery.

▶ Her breasts remain sore and tender.

▶ Mom is tired and not feeling 100 percent. Encourage her to lie down after feedings, and try to give her quiet.

NOT-TO-MISS APPOINTMENTS

▶ She might have a postsurgical checkup this week. Note: If Mom had an episiotomy, her stitches should be dissolved by the end of this week.

Family Goals

DADDY DAYCARE Take the bambino outside: In between feedings, offer to take the baby outside to the park while Mom takes a much-needed nap or gets a shower. As long as the weather isn't too cold, it's a great time to get out for a couple of minutes. Remember, the baby doesn't need to be bundled up for snow if it's only 70 degrees outside. The best rule of thumb is that a baby should have one more layer on than a normal child would need.

BROWNIE POINTS Take Mom bra shopping: If Mom is breastfeeding, chances are (unless this isn't her first child) she's realizing that she can't fit her ginormous breasts into any of her previous bras. So a family outing it is! Trying on nursing bras is a wonderful experience that is bound to bring the entire family together in a fitting room all staring at Mom's bosoms. Win–win.

Tummy Time

Depending on when your baby was born, they will have their second pediatrician's appointment at around four weeks. Remember to ask questions and to challenge the doctor if something they say doesn't feel right to you. It's important to remember that medicine is a practice, and every person, and every baby, is completely different. You are entering a world in which you will realize that throughout the baby's life, you will be this child's sole medical advocate—no one will have your child's best interests at heart more than you and your partner. You know your child best, and listening to your gut instincts about their care is very important. There are lots of theories out there about vaccination schedules, co-sleeping, breastfeeding or bottle feeding, "crying it out," and much more. Do research on your own so that you're prepared with questions and discussion points. And remember—if you don't ultimately believe that your pediatrician is the right fit, find a new one! It's very simple and shouldn't be stressful.

Getting a baby gym is a great idea. This will give your child a little bit of time to spend on their tummy, strengthening their neck muscles and practicing their kung fu grip while grabbing

BABY'S STATS

▶ Baby is ready for tummy time, which means resting on Mom or Dad's belly to work on strengthening those neck muscles.

▶ Baby may mimic facial gestures and will focus on your face.

▶ Baby is beginning to grasp.

▶ Baby may also laugh this week.

MOM'S STATS

▶ Mom's hormones are working on returning to normal.

▶ Her breasts continue to be tender.

▶ Her uterus continues to shrink, which may cause occasional bleeding or discharge.

▶ Mom may feel like she's getting the hang of things now, which can cause a lift in mood and begin to wipe away those baby blues. If they don't seem to dissipate, you need to take it upon yourself to gently continue asking about how she's feeling.

▶ Her appetite is returning to normal.

▶ Mom might feel self-conscious as she's trying to lose baby weight.

▶ Light exercise this week is great (something like walking) unless she's had a C-section or her doctor asked her to wait until her first postpartum checkup.

NOT-TO-MISS APPOINTMENTS

▶ It is time for the first four-week pediatrician's appointment.

at toys. You may actually see your baby laugh or mimic similar facial expressions as they try to focus on your face.

Mom's hormones are slowly returning to normal. If not, you'll have to pay close attention to whether Mom's emotions are evening out. Her breasts are most likely still tender, and as the uterus continues to shrink, Mom may experience bleeding or discharge. The urinary incontinence is still there, and Mom should hopefully be getting adjusted to some of the most serious sleep deprivation. As a reminder, Kegel exercises are a mom's friend and can help rebuild muscles weakened during labor and delivery. Unfortunately, that's something that you can't really help her with. Mom should consult with her physician (especially if she had a C-section), but she may have the green light to do some light exercises.

QUESTIONS TO ASK DURING THE FOUR-WEEK CHECKUP

- ▶ Does my baby weigh enough?
- ▶ Are there any skin changes to be concerned with?
- ▶ What is the vaccination schedule? What if I want to split them up one at a time or adjust the schedule?
- ▶ Is baby eating enough?
- ▶ Is baby sleeping enough?

Family Goals

BONDING TIME Take a walk: Unless Mom had a C-section, she may be cleared to get back to some light exercise, and it could be a really great idea to get outside together and take a family walk for 30 to 60 minutes at the end of the day. It will bring you together and help resume some normalcy.

DADDY DAYCARE Warm the towels: Consider warming bath towels in the dryer for when the baby comes out of the bath—what a comforting feeling!

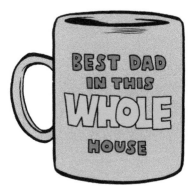

CHAPTER ELEVEN

The Eleventh Month

Chances are that you've begun to settle into a routine and you've made your way back to work in some capacity. Mom is finally beginning to feel like herself again, and that routine has certainly helped. The baby is feeding more and growing like a weed. If you're able to sleep when they sleep, you're both probably doing okay. You've had at least one if not two pediatrician's appointments. And you've noticed that your baby is beginning to communicate with you. Sure, it's still only crying and mimicking facial gestures, but it will certainly blow your mind.

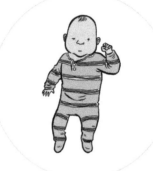

2-MONTH INFANT

AVERAGE SIZE

10 pounds

WEIGHT COMPARISON

house cat, holiday turkey

NOTES

less colicky, starting to sleep up to 6-7 hours
at a time, appetite continues to increase,
associates sights and sounds, first major
growth spurt, tummy time beginner

Hello, Smiley

This could be the week that you catch your baby smiling,
and this time it's probably not just the gas. Baby is responding
to social cues, and that reaction is genuine. The sleeping and
feeding routines may change a bit this week. The baby may be
sleeping longer at night and staying awake for longer stretches
during the day.

Your little one is growing almost one inch a week now and
is still gaining about five to seven ounces per week. They are
eating every two hours, 8 to 10 times a day, between two and
five ounces per feeding.

Mom is returning almost to her previous physical condition.
Her uterus is almost back to prepregnancy condition, and if
she's been doing Kegel exercises, the incontinence should be
tapering off. Her breasts have probably begun to normalize, and
the chapping of the nipples should start to heal. Mom should
consider sleeping when the baby sleeps if possible. I know
it's tempting to want to use that time to do things around the
house, catch up on bills, or whatever else you have going on, but
it's important to remind her that she should rest when she can.

BABY'S STATS

▶ Baby's smiles may not mean gas, but rather that they are responding to social cues.

▶ Baby recognizes and appreciates the sound of music.

▶ Baby is growing like a weed, about one inch a week.

▶ Baby is eating about every two hours, 8 to 10 times per day.

▶ Each feeding is two to five ounces per meal.

MOM'S STATS

▶ Mom is slowly returning to her normal physical condition.

▶ Doing Kegel exercises can help her gain more control of any lingering incontinence.

▶ Her breasts have started adapting to nursing, so chapping should be less of an issue now.

▶ Exercise can lessen some of her stress.

▶ For many moms, this could be the last week at home.

NOT-TO-MISS APPOINTMENTS

▶ There are no appointments unless there are complications.

Family Goals

BONDING TIME Ensure the Mom-child bond is strong: Mom should be spending as much time as possible with the baby before potentially going back to work. Make sure she is spending the majority of her time breastfeeding and bonding with the baby.

HOME CEO Hire a nanny or look into a childcare center: Spend time with your nanny (or child caretakers) and get on the same page with the feeding and sleeping schedule. If you're lucky, you may have some grandparents nearby who will be able to help!

Introducing the Bottle

If your baby is nursing and Mom is planning to return to work, this is a great week to introduce baby to the bottle. Mom can continue to pump breast milk, or you could transition to formula. Some mothers pump or nurse for a year or more, and others find it too time-consuming or painful—and to each her own. You can take a stab at feeding, which is great bonding time and also gives Mom a break. If your baby isn't necessarily receiving the new nipple with open arms, it helps to just let the nipple touch the baby's lips and allow a dribble of milk to come out—that should help in the overall introduction.

Baby's sleeping and feeding patterns are evening out, and at this point, you should be a pro at changing those diapers.

Mom is almost back to normal physically, and if this is week 6 postpartum, she will likely be given the green light to resume sexual activities, that is, if overall exhaustion and other issues aren't superseding those urges. She needs your continued support emotionally and physically, as she may become hyperfocused on her appearance around this time, given that she may be returning to work or that sex is back on the table.

BABY'S STATS

▶ Baby is consuming more at feeding time and possibly going a little bit longer between meals.

▶ Baby is keeping pace with the previous week, eating as many as 10 times a day, two to five ounces at a time. Your baby is growing almost one inch a week.

MOM'S STATS

▶ Mom's uterus has returned to normal.

▶ Mom is dropping weight, especially if she's breastfeeding.

▶ If Mom is continuing to breastfeed, her appetite may increase.

▶ Mom may be ready for sex again. She may be hyperfocused on appearance this week, especially if sex is back on the table.

▶ She may still be carrying extra weight, especially around the stomach area.

NOT-TO-MISS APPOINTMENTS

▶ This is the time for the six-week postpartum checkup for Mom. If you're going with Mom for the appointment, come up with a few questions on how you can help Mom continue to recover. Also, ask any questions that relate to specific concerns about Mom's mood and emotional well-being.

▶ Mom may be returning to work.

Fewer Crying Jags

There's some great news this week. Unless your baby has colic, you may notice that the number of crying jags has lessened. Colic is a condition marked by recurrent episodes of prolonged and uncontrollable crying for up to three hours or more of an unknown cause in an otherwise healthy infant. Don't worry; if your baby has colic, it will usually subside after three to four months. Normally, a baby should be sleeping almost six to seven hours a night at this point, which means more sleep for Mom and Dad. Creating a nighttime feeding routine will help ensure that those six to seven hours happen.

The baby is still growing about one inch and seven ounces per week, and consuming four to five ounces of milk every three to four hours. Sensory information is high on the achievement list this week, as your baby is associating sights and sounds and focusing on different objects with their eyes.

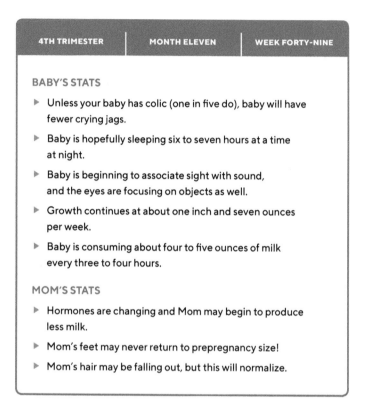

BABY'S STATS

▶ Unless your baby has colic (one in five do), baby will have fewer crying jags.

▶ Baby is hopefully sleeping six to seven hours at a time at night.

▶ Baby is beginning to associate sight with sound, and the eyes are focusing on objects as well.

▶ Growth continues at about one inch and seven ounces per week.

▶ Baby is consuming about four to five ounces of milk every three to four hours.

MOM'S STATS

▶ Hormones are changing and Mom may begin to produce less milk.

▶ Mom's feet may never return to prepregnancy size!

▶ Mom's hair may be falling out, but this will normalize.

Mom should basically be back to normal, and this week would be a great opportunity to help her resume regular workouts, including strength training and cardiovascular fitness like walking, running, or whatever she enjoyed before her pregnancy.

STICKING TO A ROUTINE

Creating a solid routine is as easy as sticking to a time line. You and your partner should make an effort to eat at about the same time every night and feed the baby about the same time every night. "Tanking up" is a phrase that refers to a heavy feeding just before lying the baby down for the night—this generally ensures a longer stretch of sleep right off the bat. A routine can also include certain music, ocean sounds, or white noise. Don't stay up too late after baby goes to bed, otherwise you'll get caught not getting enough sleep for yourself.

Family Goals

BONDING TIME Allot special time for Mom and baby: If Mom has gone back to work, make sure she is scheduling time with baby so as not to miss milestones in growth and development.

DADDY DAYCARE Spend time feeding the baby: This is a great time for Dad to practice filling and warming a bottle. Get your feeding technique down! You can also help Mom out by bagging and labeling breast milk with dates. Some will go into the refrigerator, and the rest will likely go into the freezer to beef up your surplus.

Was That Two Months Already?

Two months have flown by, and your baby is now following routines you've set, which is making life so much more manageable than it was a few weeks ago. Your baby is likely feeding about six times within a 24-hour stretch, upping the amount consumed with each passing day and week.

Growth spurts should be expected, so don't be surprised if your baby all of a sudden is crying for more food after just being fed. As for developmental milestones, it's easy for parents to compare one child to another or get focused on parameters listed within different resource publications, but it's wise not to do that. Let your doctor tell you if there's something to really be concerned with, but remember there's a wide range of what is "healthy" for babies.

Mom should be back to normal physically (unless she's still breastfeeding), as most systems have snapped back into place, which includes her period. This means she's ovulating, so be careful when reestablishing the normal routine of sex and intimacy. Unless you want to have another kid very soon, make sure that you are being careful and have birth control in place.

BABY'S STATS

▶ Learning to follow routines, your new creature is becoming a creature of habit.

▶ Baby is likely feeding about six times in 24 hours, consuming more and more in each sitting.

▶ This is a common week for a growth spurt.

▶ Baby is getting stronger and sleeping for longer stretches at night.

MOM'S STATS

▶ Most of her systems are back to normal unless she is breastfeeding.

▶ If Mom isn't breastfeeding exclusively, her period may be returning, which means she's also ovulating. Which means she can get pregnant again. Which means *be careful*.

▶ Her body is adapting to postpartum hormonal changes and may seem more on an even keel.

▶ Mom may be becoming a seasoned pro very quickly. However, every mom moves at her own pace, and it may take a little longer than some to find a rhythm.

NOT-TO-MISS APPOINTMENTS

▶ The two-month appointment for baby happens now. Most pediatricians will want to begin immunizing.

Family Goals

CONVERSATION STARTERS Talk about birth control:
With ovulation returning and sex on the table, it's
wise to talk about what your plan is moving forward.

CONVERSATION STARTERS Talk about how you want
to immunize your child: You and your partner may
want to review the immunization schedule that's recom-
mended by your pediatrician and do your own research on
each one, including looking at the side effects. My wife and
I chose an alternative schedule, choosing never to do more
than one vaccination at a time and spreading them out over
a longer period of time. Most pediatricians these days are
very open to discussing all of this.

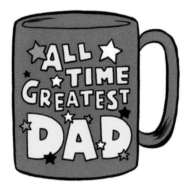

CHAPTER TWELVE

The Twelfth Month

These are the final four weeks of the fourth trimester. You and your partner may even feel like old pros at this stage of the game. You've both made it through the physically and emotionally demanding rigors of pregnancy and supported each other from the very beginning. Mom should be feeling almost normal again, and continuing to breastfeed the baby if that's what she chose to do. You've become a veteran diaper changer and bottle warmer, and your baby loves to be cuddled by Dad when it's his turn for a bottle feeding. Enjoy these first precious weeks and months of having a newborn—it sounds cliché, but they *do* grow up so fast. These are times with your son or daughter that you'll never get back again.

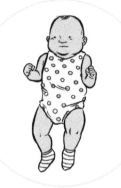

3-MONTH INFANT

AVERAGE SIZE

15 pounds

WEIGHT COMPARISON

19-inch flat screen TV, medium-sized bag of dog food

NOTES

baby is sleeping through the night (if you're lucky),
self soothes, moves from side to back during tummy time,
sucks thumbs, coos, smiles and laughs

Old Pros

As you enter your third month of parenthood, you probably feel like a seasoned pro. Mom is more than likely creeping back to her normal physical appearance, and you're both getting a decent amount of sleep. Not everyone will be on this timetable, so don't fret! Babies around the age of nine weeks are fun, too! They're animated and interactive while smiling and gurgling and laughing.

Hopefully, your baby is sleeping through the night and potentially able to self-soothe if they wake up in the middle of the night. This soothing could come in the form of music or a pacifier, or you may have a thumb sucker! You may also want to keep an extra special eye on baby during tummy time. It might be a bit early for your baby to roll over, but he can certainly go from side to back.

Mom should be feeling much better these days. She should be getting more sleep, and her pregnancy fog should be replaced with baby brain (which can really apply to both of you)—the tendency to get distracted from time to time by all of the baby's needs.

BABY'S STATS

▶ Baby may be sleeping through the night, although relapses happen.

▶ Baby is almost able to self-soothe with a pacifier or their thumb.

▶ If baby wakes up, letting them cry for a few minutes may be all they need to get back to sleep.

▶ Since baby's moving like a little worm during tummy time, more supervision could be required.

MOM'S STATS

▶ Mom may continue to nurse exclusively because it is beneficial for weight control and keeping periods at bay.

▶ Pregnancy brain has been replaced by baby brain, which means that she seems distracted by all of the baby's needs.

Family Goals

BONDING TIME Schedule a date night: If your baby is accepting the bottle, they might be ready to stay for a few hours with Grandma or another caretaker you trust. If all is going well, this might be good time for you and your partner to schedule a night out together to reconnect. Keep it low-key and local just in case you need to rush back home for the baby.

DADDY DAYCARE Focus on tummy time: With a few times on the mat every day, baby will soon be able to hold their head up and gain a whole new perspective on the world!

Double Digits

Your baby is a whopping 10 weeks old, and hopefully has their routines down pat. Naps are about an hour, give or take, and baby could take two to three per day. Your baby is eating four to six ounces every three to four hours, although the frequency or amounts may be greater when they hit a growth spurt. Your baby is also sleeping between 15 and 17 hours per day, with the bulk of that being 8 to 10 hours at night.

Mom is doing great, and her physical changes this week will be mostly attributed to her sleep, diet, and exercise, as well as to whether she is breastfeeding. Hopefully, Mom is thriving right now. However, she could still be experiencing some guilt if she feels like she's not enjoying every single moment of the baby's life. Hop on the reassurance train and give her that boost she might need. It's easy for any mom to get frustrated or overwhelmed from time to time.

Family Goals

DADDY DAYCARE Try to get baby to roll over: If baby has mastered tummy time, they might be ready to start rolling over. When you're playing on the floor with the

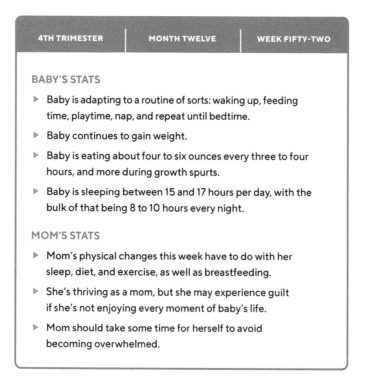

BABY'S STATS

▶ Baby is adapting to a routine of sorts: waking up, feeding time, playtime, nap, and repeat until bedtime.

▶ Baby continues to gain weight.

▶ Baby is eating about four to six ounces every three to four hours, and more during growth spurts.

▶ Baby is sleeping between 15 and 17 hours per day, with the bulk of that being 8 to 10 hours every night.

MOM'S STATS

▶ Mom's physical changes this week have to do with her sleep, diet, and exercise, as well as breastfeeding.

▶ She's thriving as a mom, but she may experience guilt if she's not enjoying every moment of baby's life.

▶ Mom should take some time for herself to avoid becoming overwhelmed.

baby, help them get used to the movements and sensation by rolling them on their back, gently of course.

 BROWNIE POINTS Insist that Mom go out: Encourage or even insist that Mom leave the nest for a bit to catch up with some girlfriends for a bite to eat. You will get some quality time with your child, and your partner will get to enjoy some of the fun times that she has been missing.

Preferences

With eating and sleeping schedules set, your baby is still gaining almost seven ounces per week and may have already grown out of some of their clothing. Your baby's personality is ever changing, and you are familiar with how your baby is communicating with coos and smiles, laughs, and giggles.

Stay on high alert these days, as this is the time of oral exploration. Your baby may be trying to gnaw or chew on anything and everything in sight.

Hopefully, Mom is in a chipper mood, continuing to exercise, getting proper sleep, and watching her diet. She might also still be losing hair that wasn't lost during the pregnancy. Don't be alarmed if the shower drain is more clogged than normal for the next few months.

Family Goals

HOME CEO Watch for choking hazards: With that age of oral exploration comes the need for being mindful about choking hazards baby may have access to. This is just a small step toward having to babyproof the entire house if you haven't done so yet!

BABY'S STATS

▶ Baby could be indicating preferences to you.

▶ Baby is familiar with your personality.

▶ Baby is cooing and smiling, and laughing at certain things and enjoying them.

▶ Baby could be growing out of clothes.

▶ Baby's sleep and eating schedule is clearly set now.

▶ Watch for baby putting everything within reach in their mouth.

MOM'S STATS

▶ As baby nears three months, Mom might start to realize just how quickly the time is going and feel a wave of nostalgia or desire to slow things down.

▶ Mom may want to buy clothes for herself (as she returns to normal weight) or the baby (who is growing!). She might also want another cool gadget, the hands-free pumping bra.

HOME CEO Come up with a plan for old clothing: Your baby will quickly grow into new sizes, and you should discuss whether you're going to donate clothes as they outgrow them or simply store them away in 30-gallon plastic bins until the next kid comes along (like we did).

The First Three Months

Only three months ago, you and your partner thought this baby would never come. Here you are, riding high with a beautiful addition to your family. Baby is still eating between five and seven ounces at a sitting and can eat on a schedule of four to five times a day. From here on out, your baby will gain about two pounds per month (give or take) until about seven years of age and will hit milestones rapidly.

Mom may be returning to work this week after being on leave. With the return could come personal conflict, worry about childcare, or just separation anxiety. All of these feelings are normal. Hopefully, Mom is also gaining confidence and settling in to enjoy her new role.

Family Goals

CONVERSATION STARTERS Discuss the when and what of solid foods: You and your partner may want to talk with your pediatrician about introducing solid foods when the baby is four to six months old. Also, you might discuss food allergies and what you can do to help prevent them.

BABY'S STATS

- ▶ Baby will gain about two pounds per month (give or take) from now until about seven months old.

- ▶ Baby is eating about five to seven ounces at every sitting.

- ▶ Baby is sleeping about 15 to 16 hours a day, and sleep times are normalizing into a routine.

MOM'S STATS

- ▶ Mom may be feeling conflict about separation if she hasn't returned to work yet.

- ▶ Mom will need to decide if she's going to pump or transition the baby to formula. If Mom is going to continue to breast-feed, consider for how long.

NOT-TO-MISS APPOINTMENTS

- ▶ Baby's next checkup and immunizations are scheduled for month 4.

FUN PROJECTS Continue to be the historian: Baby is rolling over, creeping, crawling, and walking, and these are exciting things to watch and chronicle.

HOME CEO Prepare the home for a mobile baby and high-energy toddler! Do your research and get this done—it will save you a lot of stress moving forward. Take care of things like corner bumpers for tables, electrical outlet covers, locks on the toilet lids, locks on cupboards that contain cleaners, and other issues that pose danger to a crawling, cruising, and eventually walking baby.

THE FOURTH-TRIMESTER CHECKLIST

HOME:

☐ Be prepared for visitors especially during your first weeks at home. Make sure that everyone washes their hands and disinfects!

☐ Look into hiring a nanny or enrolling your child in a child-care center. Do your homework, spend time with them, and get them on the same page with the feeding and sleeping schedule. If you are lucky enough, enlist the help of the grandparents that are nearby.

☐ Come up with a plan for old baby clothing.

☐ Prepare the home for a mobile baby and high-energy toddler.

BABY:

☐ Now is the time to use those childcare skills. Be number one at changing diapers and practice your swaddling technique.

☐ Don't forget to play with your beautiful new baby!

☐ Take the baby outside between feedings.

☐ Spend time feeding your baby and organizing and labeling breast milk.

☐ Focus on tummy time.

☐ Be the historian: be sure to record everything your baby is doing with pictures, videos, and journals.

MOM:

- ☐ Help mom with breastfeeding by educating yourself on latching techniques, types of equipment for pumping, and how to safely store breast milk.

- ☐ Be extra supportive of mom as she recovers from labor pains and watch for signs of postpartum mood disorders.

- ☐ If your partner is going back to work, make sure she is scheduling time with the baby so she is not missing milestones in growth and development.

- ☐ As soon as your baby is accepting the bottle, look into scheduling a date night.

MEDICAL APPOINTMENTS:

- ☐ Six-week postpartum checkup for mom
- ☐ For baby:
  - ☐ 3 to 5 days after birth
  - ☐ 1-month checkup
  - ☐ 2-month checkup

Conclusion

This is where I leave you, at least for now. It's been an extraordinary ride we've taken together. I hope that I've given you a decent account of each week in a pregnancy year, coupled with a few humorous stories along the way. If you decide to continue having children, perhaps my trimester checklists will serve as a foundation that you can build on—adding your own notes along the way. Each dad's journey is different, and that's what makes it beautiful.

As I sign off, I can't help but go back to that saying my wife once heard: "Women become mothers the moment they find out they're pregnant, and men become fathers when they hold their babies for the first time—but there are nine months in between." I'm a firm believer that men can feel like fathers long before they ever lay eyes on their babies. This book was created to empower us to be better partners and better versions of ourselves. Get invested in your partner's pregnancy even before day 1. And when the moment comes, be the best damn dad that you can be.

Glossary

1st stage of labor: Mom's contractions are causing her to seize up and potentially claw holes in your new button-up or the armrest of the leather recliner. Those contractions are close enough and strong enough to begin changes in her cervical dilation. This stage won't end until she's dilated to 10 centimeters.

2nd stage of labor: Cue Salt-N-Pepa because this stage may as well be called PUSH IT. The act of pushing could last anywhere from 20 minutes to three or more hours. During this stage, her contractions will begin to slow down to between two and five minutes and last as long as 1 minute to 1½ minutes. Mom will continue pushing during those contractions, which will push the baby down through the birth canal.

3rd stage of labor: A lot of parents don't recognize this stage of labor. This stage occurs immediately after the baby is born, and it consists of the delivery of the placenta. It is not as intense as the actual birth; the uterus gently contracts to release the placenta.

afterbirth: After the baby is delivered, the uterus pushes out the placenta, as well as the other membranes that Mom has held in her uterus.

amniotic fluid: The fluid that surrounds the baby while in utero. It protects the baby by acting as a bit of a shock absorber, but it also helps the lungs develop.

areola: A fun word to say publicly when you're looking to make those around you blush or feel awkward. If the nipple were the bullseye, the areola would be the rest of the circle surrounding it. Normally pinkish or brown in hue, it will likely darken throughout pregnancy, making it easier for baby to see to breastfeed.

birth plan: The plan, either written or verbally discussed with your (her) doctor, that describes how you'd like your labor and delivery to occur. It normally addresses things like pain medication, breastfeeding, and who you and your partner want in the delivery room when it's time.

Braxton Hicks: While it sounds like the lead singer of a pop band in the '80s or '90s, the only gig going on is in Mom's uterus. Braxton Hicks are contractions that start as early as the second trimester, but can also occur when Mom is overly tired or potentially after sexual intercourse. These are often referred to as "practice contractions."

breech: Normally the fetus moves toward the birth canal during the third trimester, but this doesn't always happen. Breech is when the baby has its feet or buttocks facing downward. A C-section is generally required for delivery.

cervix: The circular opening that connects the uterus to the vagina. Its dilation allows the baby to be born during labor.

cesarean section (C-section): The surgical delivery method that requires doctors to make an incision in the lower abdomen and uterus. Recovery methods and time line vary from that of natural birth.

colic: When an infant has excessive jags of crying and irritability. Generally, for a baby to be diagnosed with colic, they must cry for more than three hours a day, more than three days a week, for three weeks or more.

colostrum: The fluid produced by Mom's breasts before they actually produce milk. It's a fluid rich with protein and important antibodies that the newborn will need for nourishment during those first precious days after birth.

cord blood banking: After your baby is born, you'll have the option (you'll probably discuss this well before delivery) of collecting and storing the blood that's left in the umbilical cord and placenta. The idea is that this blood contains stem cells that could potentially be used later in life to treat medical issues with your child or someone else.

crowning: This has nothing to do with watching King Joffrey Baratheon take the throne in *Game of Thrones* but instead is the moment when you can first see your baby's head begin to emerge from Mom's vagina.

cystic fibrosis: A genetic disorder that causes thick, sticky mucus to build up in the baby's lungs and digestive tract. Genetic testing can be done ahead of time, but it's important to keep in mind that *both* parents must have the genetic mutation in order for it to be present in the child.

dilation: The gradual process by which the cervix begins to open so the baby can make its way through the birth canal.

doula: A labor coach. A doula doesn't necessarily have medical training, but she can help with emotional support during labor and delivery and offer other types of help once Mom is home with baby.

Down syndrome: A genetic abnormality. Genetic testing and screenings can be done during the first and second trimesters to determine whether or not this is something to be concerned about.

ectopic pregnancy: This occurs when the fertilized embryo attaches itself outside the uterus (most often in the fallopian tube) instead of the uterine lining. This is a threat to mom's health, and the pregnancy must be ended.

effacement: When Mom's cervix thins out during labor, allowing it to stretch so the baby can pass through during labor.

epidural: An injection into the space just outside Mom's spinal cord and serves as a method of pain relief. It lessens nerve sensitivity and blocks feeling to the lower body, but Mom stays alert during the process.

episiotomy: A cut that's made to widen the opening of Mom's vagina in the event that baby is too big to pass through naturally.

fontanel: The soft spot on an infant's skull, the space in the skull in which the bone hasn't fully fused together yet.

full term: The phrase used for the beginning of Week 39 through the end of Week 40 of pregnancy. Any baby born prior to 38 weeks and 6 days is considered premature.

fundal height: The measurement used to determine the position of the top of Mom's uterus during pregnancy.

high-risk pregnancy: A phrase used when Mom or baby is at an increased risk for health problems. This term can be use in the event of high blood pressure, multiple babies, or a mom who has crossed a certain age threshold.

lanugo: The extremely fine and very soft hair that covers a baby's body while in utero.

lightening: The period in which the baby drops or descends into Mom's pelvis. This could happen several weeks before labor or when labor begins.

lightning crotch: Sounds like fraternity-speak for someone who has it "going on" downstairs, but that's not the case here. LC is a term that refers to the sudden shooting pain that occurs in Mom's pelvis, rectum, or vulva, caused by baby's movement inside of the womb.

lochia: The initial discharge that Mom experiences after giving birth. It's composed mostly of blood and pieces of fetal membrane.

meconium: The earliest stool of an infant. Sticky and comparable to tar, it generally lasts for a few days after birth and is composed of a combination of things (such as mucus, bile, cells, lunago) ingested during baby's time in the womb.

nesting: Mom's instinctual motivation to organize and dial in the household before the baby comes. Nesting may very well have you cleaning out the garage, climbing into crawlspaces to retrieve storage bins, and ultimately amassing a stockpile of yard sale goods that takes up a bay in the garage.

preeclampsia: A disorder in which Mom has higher blood pressure than normal, as well as significant levels of protein in her urine. This condition generally occurs after 20 weeks and is something that the doctor can screen and monitor.

pregnancy brain: Sudden onset of increased forgetfulness and specifically the inability to remember where anything is at any given moment.

prolactin: A protein that enables Mom to produce milk.

restless legs syndrome: A fierce urge to move one's legs. This condition most likely won't occur on the dance floor at your company holiday party but rather in bed as Mom fights to get a solid night of sleep.

sciatica: A condition in which the baby is most likely sitting on Mom's sciatic nerve, causing a shooting pain from the lower back into one side of the leg.

swaddling: A technique or practice of tightly wrapping a baby in a muslin or another breathable blanket so as to provide the feeling of warmth and security.

tanking: The idea that you feed your baby as much as possible before bedtime, hoping that they will sleep soundly and give you and your partner more time to catch up on that much-needed rest.

Resources

AllProDad.com, All Pro Dad

AtHomeDad.org, National At-Home Dad Network

BabyCenter.com, BabyCenter

CityDadsGroup.com, City Dads Group

Dad.info, DAD.info

Dad2Summit.com, The Dad 2.0 Summit

DadOrAlive.com, *Dad or Alive*

DaddyStyleDiaries.com, *Daddy Style Diaries*

DesignerDaddy.com, *Designer Daddy*

Fatherhood.org, National Fatherhood Initiative

Fatherly.com, *Fatherly*

Fathers.com, National Center for Fathering

Healing Hearts (Baby Loss Comfort): BabyLossComfort.com/grief-resources

HowToBeADad.com, *HowToBeADad*

LifeOfDad.com, Life of Dad

Loss Advisors Loss Doulas:
BabyLossFamilyAdvisors.org/parent-services.html

LunchboxDad.com, *Lunchbox Dad*

MrDad.com, Mr. Dad

NationalShare.org, Share: Pregnancy & Infant Loss Support

Postpartum.net, Postpartum Support International

PostpartumDads.org, PostpartumDads

PostpartumProgress.com, *Postpartum Progress*

TheDadWebsite.com, The Dad Website

References

Borgenicht, Louis, and Joe Borgenicht. *The Baby Owner's Manual*. Philadelphia: Quirk Books, 2012.

Brott, Armin A., and Jennifer Ash. *The Expectant Father*. New York: Abbeville Press, 2015.

Greenberg, Gary, and Jeannie Hayden. *Be Prepared*. New York: Simon & Schuster, 2004.

Jones, Sandy, and Marcie Jones, with Michael Crocetti. *Great Expectations: Baby's First Year*. New York: Sterling, 2007.

Mactavish, Scott. *The New Dad's Survival Guide*. New York: Little, Brown and Company, 2005.

Murkoff, Heidi, and Sharon Mazel. *What to Expect When You're Expecting*. New York: Workman Publishing, 2016.

Pfeiffer, John. *Dude, You're Gonna Be a Dad!* Avon: MA: Adams Media, 2011.

Watson, Benjamin. *The New Dad's Playbook*. Grand Rapids, MI: Baker Books, 2017.

Index

Acknowledgments

Without my wife, Jen, and our three children, Ava, Charlie, and Mason (with baby girl coming soon), I'd be in no position to even begin writing a book like this. My love and gratitude extends to them all—they make every day an adventure, full of laughter and love.

To my parents, Bruce and Joan, who raised three boys and helped me become the man and father I am today—I'm forever grateful.

To my brothers, Eric and Travis, who might one day decide to settle down and start families of their own, you may benefit from these musings and I wish you only the very best.

To the extended Kulp family, Bob and Elaine Mayer and the Mayer, Hellwig, and Trost families—thanks for always being there with a warm heart and never-ending support.

About the Author

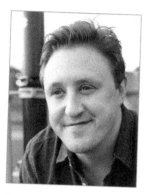

Adrian Kulp has worked as a comedy booking agent for CBS late-night television, as an executive for Adam Sandler's Happy Madison Productions, and as a vice president of development for Chelsea Handler's Borderline Amazing Productions.

For the past eight years, he's been the voice behind the popular dad blog turned parenting memoir *Dad or Alive: Confessions of an Unexpected Stay-at-Home Dad*. He's produced the reality series *Modern Dads* for A&E Networks, is a regular contributor to *HuffPost*, *The Bump*, and *Parents* magazine, and is a partner at the massive online fatherhood community, *Life of Dad*.

He lives on the coast in Suffolk, Virginia, with his wife, Jen, and their three kids, Ava, Charlie, and Mason, and they have another baby girl on the way.